ARE YOU LOOKING FOR A BRAIN BOOST?

- You can't remember dates and places?
- Names of people you know well slip your mind?
- You sometimes can't remember what you were doing?
- You find it difficult to stay focused?
- You can't remember phone numbers as you used to?
- You're afraid it's Alzheimer's?
- You wish you had more energy?
- Your circulation isn't what it used to be?
- You're worried that your mind and body are failing?

**FIND OUT HOW GINKGO
AND OTHER NATURAL MEMORY
ENHANCERS CAN GIVE YOUR BRAIN
AND YOUR HEALTH A BOOST**

GINKGO

NATURE'S BRAIN BOOSTER

Alan H. Pressman, D.C., Ph.D., C.C.N.

with Helen Tracy

Produced by The Philip Lief Group, Inc.

AN AVON BOOK

The ideas, procedures, and suggestions in this book are intended to supplement, not replace, the medical advice of a trained medical professional. All matters regarding your health require medical supervision. Consult your physician before adopting the suggestions in this book, as well as about any condition that may require diagnosis or medical attention. The authors and publisher disclaim any liability arising directly or indirectly from the use of this book.

AVON BOOKS, INC.
1350 Avenue of the Americas
New York, New York 10019

Copyright © 1999 by The Philip Lief Group, Inc.
Published by arrangement with The Philip Lief Group, Inc.
Library of Congress Catalog Card Number: 98-91017
ISBN: 0-380-80640-1
www.avonbooks.com/wholecare

First Wholecare Printing: June 1999

AVON WHOLECARE TRADEMARK REG. U.S. PAT. OFF. AND IN OTHER COUNTRIES, MARCA REGISTRADA, HECHO EN U.S.A.

Printed in the U.S.A.

WCD 10 9 8 7 6 5 4 3 2 1

**To Howard Smith, who never
forgets the important things.**

Special thanks to Isis M. Medina, D.C., M.S.,
New York City College of Chiropractic;
Sara Thompson, M.S., San Diego State University;
Diane Epstein, M.S., M.F.A.; Kathy Clayton and
Karen Creviston, Timberland Library System,
Amanda Park Branch; and the staffs of
Northwestern University Library
and University of Washington Library.

Contents

Introduction

A college student walks into a final exam. Her grade point average is on the line, which means that her chances of getting into a good graduate school are riding, like a monkey, on her back. She has studied for weeks, reviewing the material again and again, and she went over all of it again last night. She knows it. But will she remember it?

A middle-aged business executive sits at a meeting. Around him are young movers and shakers, sharp as a tack and twice as bright. He has a presentation to make, complete with slides, charts, and all the aids technology can give him. But what can help him remember all the information he's going to need to answer questions from all those young MBAs?

A woman in her sixties stands at the door to her suburban home. For the past 20 minutes she has been looking for her car keys. Now, already late for the session she's supposed to teach in the library literacy program, she is near tears with frustration and, yes, fear. Is her memory going?

The quest for something that will improve memory has been going on for thousands of years. Today, however, there is an urgency to it that seems to result from the pace and pressure of the modern lifestyle. With the rise of technology, the human brain is being pushed to its limits, and many of us feel the need to try to go beyond those limits. Just as we buy equipment to make our bodies stronger and more efficient, we are now looking for something to make the same kind of improvement in our minds. In a world where competition is fierce and apparently unrelenting, we are looking for a competitive edge.

And there are hundreds of companies out there offering quick fixes that sound possible, promising, and sometimes miraculous. The question is: Do any of these drugs, herbs, and potions work? Is there really a substance that will make the little gray cells stand up and take notice? Or are we being sold a bill of goods, as we so often have been, with regard to our physical health?

The latest substance to attract our attention is also one of the oldest. Ginkgo biloba has a history that stretches back for centuries, even millennia. It may be the newest "wonder cure," but it has been around for longer than most of the drugs we take without thinking twice. During that time, it has been proven to be remarkably safe. In addition, it's not prohibitively expensive. But does it work? What can it do? Those are the questions— among others—that this book was written to answer.

Why is everyone talking about ginkgo biloba?

That question can be answered with one acronym—JAMA. The bible of the medical establishment is a periodical called the *Journal of the American Medical Association*. In its pages are reported the most important medical advances, the most promising new treatments and medications, the best hopes for the future of medicine. But JAMA does not publish every research study done in every small university. It is conservative and cautious and very picky. That's why articles that *do* get published in the journal are paid attention to—by scientists, doctors, and the media.

On October 22, 1997, JAMA published an article with this imposing title: "A placebo-controlled, double-blind randomized trial of an extract of ginkgo biloba for dementia." What it amounted to was that a group of researchers, headed by Pierre L. LeBars, had taken 309 people in the early stages of Alzheimer's disease and given them tests to measure their memories. Then, after a year of taking either ginkgo or a placebo, the patients were tested again. The patients didn't know who was taking which pill and neither did the researchers. It was a good, objective, and scientifically respectable study. And its results were clear. The people who took ginkgo did better than the people who didn't.

This "incredible breakthrough" was reported on news shows and in newspapers throughout the country. Next to a cure for cancer, a treatment for Alzheimer's was probably the biggest medical news most people could imagine. Suddenly, everyone was talking about ginkgo biloba.

What exactly did the study show?

Put simply, a significant number of the people taking ginkgo had no additional loss of their memory functions during the year of the study and, in fact, experienced *measurable improvement*. We'll go further into the exact parameters of the research later, but suffice it to say that in this, the first study of ginkgo and Alzheimer's done in the United States, the herb performed. It seemed to indicate some reason for hopefulness among sufferers.

What was the public's reaction to the study?

There was a great deal of excitement, of course. Sales of ginkgo had been climbing for the last several years because of word of mouth and the results of studies done in other countries. But when the JAMA article came out, they shot through the roof. Companies that sell ginkgo rushed onto the Internet and into print with claims that the ancient Chinese herb could "cure Alzheimer's." They went further, in fact, to declare that ginkgo was a memory enhancer that could help college students pass tests, shoppers do without grocery lists, and businesspeople walk out of conference rooms with whole meetings imprinted on their brains.

This reaction was encouraged by the media. In recent years, the networks and wire services have been watching JAMA like hawks, searching for "medical breakthroughs" and "scientific miracles." Their reportage of news regarding health and medicine has tended increasingly toward the sensational, and it has become more and more difficult to find balanced accounts. Unfortunately, this often leads to false hopes. Another result, almost as serious, is that some people become skeptical and begin to ignore all news of new discoveries.

What was the medical establishment's reaction to the study?

Doctors were cautious. Some were impatient, and a few were downright hostile. That is not surprising, given the media blitz on the subject. Many doctors probably felt, instinctively, that they needed to provide balance by coming down on the negative side of the question. This was certainly the position taken by the Alzheimer's Association, a national group dedicated to promoting education and research concerning the disease. The head of its medical advisory board, Steven DeKosky, M.D, found himself very busy going on TV shows, such as *Good Morning, America*, to say, in essence, "Don't stop taking your medication and switch to ginkgo. We don't know enough yet." On *Nightline*, it was Steven Ferris, M.D., who carried the banner for caution. (Both doctors, by the way, are consultants for pharmaceutical companies.) That was also the reaction of a lot of general practitioners and geriatric specialists. We talked to doctors while researching this book who said that they were getting dozens of patients every day who, without consulting them or any other physician, had started taking ginkgo to treat everything from absentmindedness to serious, even life-threatening illnesses.

Other medical professionals were more positive about ginkgo and its possibilities. They defended the study and JAMA for publishing it. Derrick DeSilva, M.D., who has long used herbal medicines with his patients, said, "The pioneers take all the arrows, and this is a pioneering study in this country."

So, who's right?

As you might guess, the answer doesn't lie at either of these extremes. Indeed, this kind of polarization makes it more difficult than it should be to get to the truth. But that's what we're going to try to do in this book. We'll look not only at the LeBars study and its implications but also at the long history of ginkgo as a medicinal herb in traditional medicine. This is not a drug created last year in a laboratory, but a substance that has been used for centuries by a large part of the civilized world. There is much, much more to know about it than the results of one study done in New York, no matter how interesting it was.

Was this the first important study done on ginkgo?

Far from it. Ginkgo is one of the most researched substances in the world. In the past 30 years, it has been the subject of more than 280 published studies done in Europe, especially in France and Germany, as well as in Asia and the United States.

It is currently the number one prescription in Germany. And it is the herbal medicine most frequently prescribed by physicians worldwide. These physicians do not prescribe ginkgo to their patients exclusively or even primarily for the treatment of Alzheimer's disease. It has a number of other highly important uses we will go into later.

Does anyone really know whether ginkgo works?

Yes. We know it works in a number of ways and for a number of conditions. It is an effective anti-inflammatory, like aspirin, Advil, and the steroids such as cortisone. It increases the elasticity of blood vessels throughout the body and works to prevent excessive clotting of the blood by inhibiting platelet aggregation. It is a powerful antioxidant, helping to rid the body of free radicals, which are implicated in many diseases and in the process of aging. All of these properties have been proven. What else it may do and to what extent each of its proven properties is effective in matters of memory, dementia, or any other condition is what we're going to try to explain later in this book.

Can't my doctor tell me what I need to know about ginkgo?

Some doctors could, and consulting your doctor is an important step before taking any kind of medication. However, information about ginkgo has been coming out so quickly, and in such quantity, that only a doctor with a special interest in herbal medicines is likely to be completely informed about its properties and possibilities. Your health is ultimately your responsibility, and being well informed about any treatments that may be useful to you in maintaining your health is part of that responsibility. Information enables you to ask your doctor the right questions and work with him or her to come to the right decisions. At this point in history, ginkgo biloba extract is not an accepted part of most American doctors' medicinal repertoire, but it might very well be in a few years, just as it already is in Europe. Why shouldn't you and your doctor be in the forefront of any such development?

But wouldn't the wide acceptance of an herbal medicine by the Western medical establishment be unprecedented?

Let us tell you the story of willow bark. For centuries, even millennia, the bark of the willow was used to make teas and potions to treat people all over the world. It was a staple of herbal medicine, whether practiced by old women in the forests of Europe or shamans in the woods of North America. Then, in the late nineteenth century, a German pharmaceutical company launched a program to extract the active ingredient of willow bark and to begin marketing it as a pill. In 1899, Bayer began selling the medicine, which it called aspirin (acetylsalicylic acid), and the rest, as they say, is history.

This striking example is only one of thousands. The fact is that most medicines accepted and used by the Western medical establishment are derived at some point from plants. Antibiotics are made from mold. Virtually all narcotics were originally made from the *papaver*, or poppy, which is also the source of a number of "recreational drugs," such as heroin. The crucial heart medicine digitalis is derived from the lovely foxglove. Most muscle relaxants are made from the legendary curare plant, source of the poison used by South American archers and fictional murderers. Vincristine, a medicine used to treat acute leukemia, is made from the Madagascar periwinkle. The acceptance of an extract of ginkgo biloba as a part of the medicinal repertoire would be far from unprecedented. Indeed, it would be almost boringly predictable. At this point, however, there is nothing boring about its possibilities and the benefits it may have for the health of your mind and body.

Chapter 1

Ginkgo Biloba

Although you may have heard of it only recently, ginkgo biloba is probably the world's leading over-the-counter product, with global sales that exceed two billion U.S. dollars every year. In Europe, consumers spend hundreds of millions of dollars annually for this ancient herb, and its sales in the United States are rising at a dizzying speed. In 1996, they topped $100 million, and the owner of the 140 Great Earth stores in this country reports that ginkgo sales rose 28% in 1997. Another firm reported its sales up by 32% and expected them to double in 1998. In November of 1997, the first International Ginkgo Seminar opened in Beijing under the joint sponsorship of the Chinese State Science and Technology Commission and two major international pharmaceutical companies. More than 150 scientists from research institutes and pharmaceutical laboratories attended.

This remarkable burgeoning of interest in a traditional Chinese medicinal herb raises many

questions. Some herbalists and proponents of natural medicine say it's about time American medicine paid attention to this potent, multipurpose,
nontoxic medicinal herb that has been so well received and widely used in other parts of the world.
It's difficult not to see their point.

What is ginkgo biloba?

To begin with, it's a tree, otherwise known as the
maidenhair tree or Bai Guo. As one of the gym-
nosperms (pines, cedars, firs), it's virtually iden-
tical to trees that we know only from fossil rem-
nants. The last surviving member of the
Ginkgoaceae family, the ginkgo biloba tree seems
to have endured on the planet for more than 200
million years, making it the oldest species of tree
in the world.

Even the name of this remarkable tree is unusual. Its genus name, ginkgo, comes from the
Japanese name for the "fruit" of the tree, which is
really a seed. The Japanese based their name on
the Chinese ideographs "yin kuo" meaning "silver
fruit." Its species name, biloba, is from the Latin,
meaning two-lobed, which refers to the unusual
shape of its leaf. Topping a long, slender stalk, the
leaf is divided into two graceful lobes which together look something like a fan. It is called
"maidenhair tree," because the leaves resemble
those of the maidenhair fern, and "Tree of 40
Gold Crowns," because the leaves turn a striking
gold in the fall. Ginkgo is the only tree now living
that is known to produce motile sperm cells,

which are characteristic of lower orders of plants, such as ferns, and are evidence of its prehistoric origins.

During the Mesozoic Era, two seed trees arose from the collapse of the Coal Age, just missing extinction. They are still around. One is the sago palm, a cycad. About the only place you'll find it is in a botanical garden. The other is the ginkgo. These two spread across the newly formed continents virtually unchecked. Without any real competition, they established themselves all over the world and for millions of years were the dominant plant life. The period is sometimes called the Age of Cycads, when it is not being called the Age of Reptiles because of those rather large creatures who lived among the cycads and ginkgoes.

The sole limitation on the cycads and ginkgoes, as well as the ferns and mosses that were their contemporaries, was that they could reproduce only in areas where there was a lot of moisture, because the trees' seeds were fertilized by swimming male cells, as were the spores of the ferns and mosses. The cycads and ginkgoes were transitional plants between those that reproduced by spores and those that reproduced by seed—half one and half the other.

In the words of Wayne Armstrong of Palomar College, ginkgo is a living survivor of "an ancient flora that dates back to the days of the dinosaurs. In fact, leaf imprints resembling the present-day maidenhair tree [ginkgo biloba] have been found abundantly in sedimentary rocks of the Jurassic

and Triassic Periods [135–210 million years ago]
when dinosaurs roamed the earth."

What does the ginkgo biloba tree look like?

It can grow to a height of about 130 feet. Its trunk
is slender until the tree is about 100 years old, and
then it can thicken considerably. The ginkgo's
wood is light, brittle, yellowish in color and not
particularly useful. The trunk is deeply furrowed
and highly ridged. The twigs are tan to light-gray
and often highly reflective in the winter sun. In
the spring, the ginkgo's leaves are chartreuse, and
in the fall they turn that lovely gold we mentioned
before.

Where does the tree grow now?

The ginkgo biloba tree used to grow in most
parts of the earth, as we said. With the Ice Age,
however, it disappeared from Europe, North
America, and much of Asia, remaining only in
China, where it was saved from extinction because
it was revered by Buddhist monks and planted
near temples. At least two of these stands sur-
vived. There are magnificent specimens, reputed
to be over a thousand years old, in Buddhist
temple grounds.

Its continued existence was unknown to most
of the world until a surgeon employed by the
Dutch East India Company discovered the tree in
1690. The surgeon, E. Kaempfer, who was also a
botanist, published a description of the tree in
1712, including drawings of the foliage and

"fruit." The tree was introduced into Europe before 1730, being first planted in the Botanic Garden at Utrecht. Most of the early trees raised on the Continent and in Britain appear to have been males, and De Candolle discovered the first recorded female tree near Geneva in 1814.

The ginkgo tree is now grown around the world. It was brought to North America about half a century after it was introduced in Europe, in 1784. It was first planted in the United States in a garden near Philadelphia. Every ginkgo tree, in every country, is a descendant of the stands discovered in China in the eighteenth century.

Why has the ginkgo tree survived when others haven't?

Very simply, it knows how to adapt. Indeed, the ginkgo tree is so adaptable that it can survive air pollution that chokes most other trees, as well as a variety of weather and soil conditions. This ability is probably derived from its unusual phylogenetic makeup, and it's one of the reasons that the ginkgo has become popular in so many places.

Is this the same ginkgo that's sold as an ornamental shrub?

Yes, it is. Again, its adaptability makes it highly desirable as a landscape element. However, we don't recommend going out into the yard and chewing on the leaves. All you're likely to get out of that is a stomachache. The process of extraction—from leaves to dietary supplement—is long and complicated, producing a potent and balanced substance.

What part of the ginkgo tree is used as a medicine?

Chinese medicine has traditionally used the "fruit," which is actually not a fruit at all but the kernel, or seed. The ginkgo tree is always either female or male. The female produces this fleshy fruit. The Chinese process the fruit to make a medicine that they use for asthma and other illnesses. Without such processing, it can be toxic. However, about three decades ago, European scientists began experimenting with the leaves of the tree, and the substance that is used most often as medicine comes from those leaves. It, too, requires considerable processing before it is effective as a medicine.

How long has ginkgo been used as medicine?

Ginkgo has been used in China since at least 2800 B.C. and in other Asian countries for centuries. In fact, it has been an extremely important part of the Eastern pharmaceutical repertoire, used for a variety of conditions, along with the equally important ginseng.

However, although the tree has been a familiar sight in Europe and America for some time, the herbal extract has not been significant in Western medicine. Until recently, if you looked up ginkgo in an encyclopedia, you would have found information about the tree as an ornamental plant, with no mention of its medicinal properties. Only within about the last 30 years has it become a popular herbal medicine in Europe, especially France and Germany. In Germany, it is a prescription medication and, indeed, is the most prescribed medication in that country.

What has ginkgo been used for?

It has been used for a remarkable number of conditions and illnesses. Traditionally, it was used primarily for asthma and various problems of the brain. A recent review of the Internet, however, found the herb being recommended for all of the following:

- The early stages of Alzheimer's disease
- Memory loss associated with aging
- Impotence
- Poor circulation
- Long-term therapy for stroke
- Tinnitus
- Hearing loss
- Depression in the elderly
- Asthma
- Intermittent claudication
- Vertigo
- Vascular headache
- Sensitivity to cold
- Raynaud's disease
- Diabetic tissue damage
- Inner-ear disturbances.

How could one substance help people with so many different conditions?

In the first place, we don't know yet that it can. Many studies have been done, but additional research is now in the process and should tell us considerably more. However, even what we know now makes it clear that it is quite possible ginkgo could favorably affect a wide variety of diseases and conditions.

The three *known* ways in which the herb works—as an anti-inflammatory, as an antioxidant, and as an aid to blood circulation—could have benefits for a number of medical problems. Just from the previous list, for example, half of the conditions listed—including impotence, tinnitus, memory loss, vascular headache, and intermittent claudication—might be improved by increased blood circulation. Indeed, one of the most important studies of ginkgo concerned intermittent claudication, a condition in which the sufferer loses the ability to walk for any length of time because of pain in the muscles of the legs. The problem is caused by arterial circulatory disturbances. By increasing circulation, ginkgo was found to greatly improve the ability of the patients in the study to walk distances without pain.

Ordinarily, so many different claims for one herbal medicine would be a warning sign that the information was being puffed up out of all proportion. However, ginkgo biloba may very well be one of those substances, like aspirin, that has a limited number of powers but an almost unlimited number of applications.

How does ginkgo increase blood circulation?

Actually, ginkgo boosts circulation in two ways. First, it inhibits the tendency of platelets in the blood to clump by counteracting a substance called PAF, or Platelet Aggregation Factor. Platelets, of course, are the blood cells responsible for clotting. Second, ginkgo increases the elasticity of the blood vessels, making them able to expand more easily. Simply put, ginkgo makes your blood thinner and the passages through which it flows more flexible. By doing these two things, the herbal extract makes it possible for more blood to flow through your blood vessels to areas where there might be problems, such as the lower extremities and the brain. This has important implications for memory and other cognitive functions. Just how important, we are only beginning to find out.

What do the anti-inflammatory properties of ginkgo do?

Inflammation is a local response to cell injury in the body. The injury can be caused by trauma, infection, or any of a number of other things. Inflammation is characterized by swelling, infiltration by white blood cells, heat, and pain. It is, in one sense, a beneficial response by the body to injury, in that it controls damage and eliminates damaged tissue. On the other hand, unchecked inflammation can cause serious problems. It is implicated in arthritis, for example, as well as asthma and other painful conditions. An anti-inflammatory substance, obviously, fights against inflammation. For most of this century, aspirin has been the most popular anti-inflammatory drug. Ibuprofen is another. Not all pain relievers are anti-inflammatories, however. Acetaminophen, for example, is not. One of the primary uses of steroids is anti-inflammatory.

Ginkgo is a potent anti-inflammatory substance. This property is involved in several of the purposes for which the herb has traditionally been used, as well as many of its newer uses. One of the advantages ginkgo has over other anti-inflammatories, especially the steroids, is that it has virtually no side effects. It does not, for example, cause the stomach distress that aspirin can.

What do the antioxidant properties of ginkgo do?

You've probably been hearing the word *antioxidant* a lot lately. The discovery of *free radicals* and the damage they do has made the search for effective weapons against them a priority in medical and nutritional circles. Antioxidants are those weapons. To understand what they are and what they do, we have to begin with the free radical itself.

A free radical is a molecule in which one of the electrons has been lost. When that happens, the molecule goes nuts trying to find another electron. It will rob that electron from anywhere, thereby causing damage to proteins in your healthy cells, cellular DNA, and cell membranes.

When the free radical does that, there are three possibilities. The cell may die or it may begin to grow uncontrollably, forming a tumor, or it may be repaired by an antioxidant. The damage done by free radicals is now implicated in the aging process and approximately 60 degenerative diseases. Those diseases are big ones. They include Alzheimer's, arthritis, cancer, cataracts, Parkinson's disease, phlebitis, rheumatism, and stroke, as well as less serious conditions such as varicose veins and hemorrhoids.

Where do free radicals come from?

Free radicals are produced in the body by the normal metabolic process, and there are also natural antioxidant enzymes in the body to deal with them. These enzymes graciously donate electrons to the needy free radicals, and everyone is happy. However, free radicals are also produced by air pollution, alcohol, pesticides, smoking, and other realities of modern life. The body's antioxidant enzymes require reinforcements to deal with all that. Among the antioxidant substances we now know we can enlist in the battle are glutathione (see my book, *Glutathione: The Ultimate Antioxidant*, St. Martin's Press, 1997); a number of vitamins—including A, C, and E; the minerals selenium and magnesium; a substance found in red wine; and certain components of tea. And ginkgo biloba.

How long have we known that ginkgo was all these things—an anti-inflammatory and antioxidant and an aid to blood circulation?

To answer that, let's look at one of the conditions ginkgo has been used for in Eastern medicine for thousands of years—asthma. Asthma might be described as an overreaction on the part of the respiratory system to irritants, many of which may be relatively harmless. When "attacked" by pollen, mold, or even perfume, asthmatic lungs go into defense mode. They become inflamed, which is the body's response to damage. Of course, the lungs are not being damaged by the smell of Shalimar, whatever the aesthetic response may be. Instead, it is the body's defense that becomes the problem. As a result, one part of modern asthma therapy involves using steroids to reduce the inflammation that shuts off air passages and causes asthma sufferers to gasp for air. Traditional Chinese medicine has used the anti-inflammatory ginkgo for the same purpose, whether or not the mechanism involved was known or named.

Ginkgo has also been used for a very long time to aid the circulation of the blood, a process that is somewhat more obvious in its mechanics than inflammation. The herb's antioxidant properties, however, are a new discovery, largely because free radicals are so recent an addition to our understanding of the body and its processes.

What form of ginkgo is used as a medicine in Europe and America?

The form of ginkgo used in virtually all studies is an extract of the leaves called EGb 761. Developed by European scientists, it is produced in a 15-step process that requires a 50-to-1 ratio—in terms of weight—of leaves to extract. There are dozens of other forms of ginkgo on the market today, but their efficacy has not been tested.

What are the active ingredients of this extract?

The active ingredients of EGb 761 are bio-flavonoids, such as kaempferol, quercetin, and isorhamnetine; terpene lactones, mostly ginkgo-lides (A, B, C, and M) and bilobalide; and organic acids. The ginkgolides were first isolated in 1932 by the scientist Furukawa. Their chemical structure was elucidated and named by Nakanishi in 1966. They are described by the American Botanical Council as "extremely complex molecules unique to ginkgo." The various ginkgolides differ in potency, the most active of them being Ginkgolide B. They are involved in inhibiting platelet clumping and, therefore, blood clotting.

It is important that these ingredients be balanced in the extract, and that is one reason that the standard extraction process is important. EGb 761 contains 24% flavone glycosides and 6% terpenoids, in particular ginkgolides and bilobalide. If, after reading this book, you decide to take ginkgo biloba, this is the information you should look for on the label of any brand you contemplate buying.

Are there any negative side effects to ginkgo biloba?

That is one of the remarkable things about this herb. It is extremely safe. There are almost no problems associated with taking it, and what problems there are tend to be minor. Fewer than 1% percent of patients in the clinical studies have complained of gastrointestinal upset, and those upsets were mild. Some patients who have problems with blood flow to the brain find that they have mild, transient headaches for the first few days. These go away shortly. There are no known interactions with drugs. The German Commission E guidelines list no contraindications to use during pregnancy or lactation, but I'd suggest checking with your doctor before taking it if you're pregnant.

However, people who have bleeding disorders should not take ginkgo. People who are taking blood thinners for heart conditions should have their physicians adjust their dosage if they begin taking ginkgo. Otherwise, since ginkgo further thins the blood, problems could arise for these people. There are some anecdotes in the literature concerning low blood pressure. Even though problems have not turned up in formal studies, it makes sense that people with low blood pressure should at least consult with their doctors and monitor their blood pressure. Otherwise, ginkgo is amazingly safe.

That is the basic information you need to know about ginkgo. The next chapter will deal with the herb's apparently remarkable effects on the brain and cognition.

Chapter 2

Ginkgo and Alzheimer's Disease

The recent studies about ginkgo biloba and Alzheimer's disease have caused considerable excitement and controversy. This is understandable, considering how frightening the illness is to most of us and how widespread it is becoming. If ginkgo can actually mitigate some of the nightmare aspects of the disease, it will be a tremendous boon to a large portion of our older population and to the people who care about and care for them. Only in the last few years have there been any medications at all that helped sufferers from the disease, and at least one of those medications has serious possible side effects. So far, there are no treatments for Alzheimer's that promise to cure the disease or reverse its progress.

For all our fears of Alzheimer's and our concerns about the possibility of suffering from it or watching our loved ones lose the use of their most precious faculties, it is amazing how little most of us really know about this disease. We have a general idea that it's something that makes old people forgetful, the scientific equivalent of senility. The reality is much more complex, and much more serious, than that.

What is Alzheimer's disease?

Alzheimer's disease (AD) was first identified in 1907 by a German physician named Alois Alzheimer. Obviously, the condition was named for its discoverer. It is an incurable, degenerative disease of the brain that usually occurs in the later years of life. Gradual changes in nerve cells result, over time, in loss of the ability to remember, think, reason, and coordinate movement. An ironic footnote is that these abilities are lost in reverse order to that in which they were originally acquired in childhood and in about the same length of time.

Do more people have AD than ever before?

Yes, unfortunately, they do. However, this is in part because people are living longer. The average life span of an American in 1900 was 47 years. Today, it is more than 75 years. There are now far more people in this country who fall into the age range most at risk for Alzheimer's. And so, as you would expect, far more people have it. At least half the people in nursing homes in this country have Alzheimer's disease or a related disorder. In 1998, there were about four million people in the United States who were sufferers of Alzheimer's disease. It is estimated that, by the middle of the coming century, if no cure is found, 14 million will be afflicted with the debilitating effects of this devastating disease.

Who are the people most affected by AD?

Alzheimer's usually strikes people who are over 65, although it can begin earlier. The disease is not uncommon in people in their forties and fifties and has even been detected, in rare cases, in people who are in their thirties. People who develop Alzheimer's before 65 are said to be suffering from early-onset Alzheimer's, which may be genetically different from the more common version. Women are more likely to get Alzheimer's than men are, and their susceptibility increases with age. Estimates are that 8 to 10% of all people over 65 in this country have Alzheimer's, and 30 to 45% of those over 85 have the disease. This is a remarkably large group. There are also a great many undiagnosed cases, which are revealed when public health agencies do community surveys.

In addition to age, a person's heredity can be a primary risk factor. Some studies indicate that, by the age of 90, 50% of the people who have an immediate relation with Alzheimer's will develop the disease themselves. It has been discovered that genetic mutations on chromosomes 1, 14, and 21 cause early-onset Alzheimer's. An irregularity on chromosome 19 is associated with the more common form of Alzheimer's.

In some way that is not yet clear, lack of education is also a risk factor. The percentage of people who get Alzheimer's is considerably higher among those with little education than it is among those who have, for example, college degrees. This is, of course, a difficult finding to interpret. Do people with college degrees use their brains more in their jobs, for example, and does use of the brain help to keep it healthy? Or is there some socioeconomic factor, such as nutrition, at work? More research is needed.

The other primary sufferers of Alzheimer's are those who do not have the disease themselves but devote large parts of their lives to caring for victims. The families of Alzheimer's patients carry terrible emotional, social, and financial burdens, sometimes for decades. They may risk their own health in trying to preserve the health of their loved ones. Caring for an Alzheimer's patient is one of the most stressful, heartbreaking jobs imaginable.

How does the prevalence of Alzheimer's affect all of us?

Simply, society loses a contributing member and gains one who drains the resources of not only his or her family but also the entire community. In addition, the person who has the principal responsibility for caring for the Alzheimer's sufferer may also be removed from the position of productive community member. Two people who might have been scout leaders, charity fundraisers, music teachers, artists, or civic leaders are instead caught in a tangle of physical and emotional problems from which there is, as yet, no escape but death.

What are the material costs of AD?

They are enormous. In 1985, the annual cost of caring for individuals with Alzheimer's disease and related dementias, in institutional and community settings, was estimated as between $24 billion and $48 billion. This is for direct costs alone. It is certainly considerably higher today. The consensus statement of the American Association for Geriatric Psychiatry, the Alzheimer's Association, and the American Geriatrics Society, issued in 1997, estimated current costs at about $100 billion per year. On an individual level, care for one Alzheimer's patient averages about $36,000 per year.

This estimate does not count the costs of caring for the caregiver. Up to half of primary caregivers to Alzheimer's patients develop significant psychological problems. Others suffer physically from the stress.

Who pays these costs?

Everyone does. Alzheimer's is painfully and often cripplingly expensive for the family of the patient. It also puts a terrible burden on the Medicare and Medicaid systems and other public agencies responsible for the welfare of aged citizens. And it calls on the resources of private insurers to a degree that affects the health care costs of all of us.

What causes AD?

No one knows for sure. If we did, we'd have a much better chance of combating the disease. We are, however, making progress. In the past few years, researchers have discovered, through autopsy, two sorts of abnormalities that are present in the brains of Alzheimer patients. They are *neurofibrillary tangles* and *neuritic plaques*.

Neurofibrillary tangles are found inside the hippocampus, which is the center of memory in the brain. They are tangled nerve-cell fibers. Inside each of these tangles is a protein called *tau*. The tau protein normally functions in assembling the nerve cell "skeleton." Neurofibrillary tangles have abnormal tau proteins, and it is thought the result is an error in the stability and shape of the skeleton. Neurofibrillary tangles are very rarely found in healthy brains.

Neuritic plaques are patches containing a sticky protein called *beta amyloid*. They are surrounded by dying neurons, possibly because beta amyloid causes a narrowing of blood vessels in the brain. The loss of blood to the cells kills them. Again, neuritic plaques are not found in healthy brains.

The result of neurofibrillary tangles and neuritic plaques seems to be massive nerve-cell death and therefore loss of brain function. Having said that, we are only one step closer to the answer because we don't yet know what causes the neurofibrillary tangles and neuritic plaques. However, some very important speculations are being made regarding viruses, chemical neurotransmitters, chemical toxins in the environment, immune system deficiencies, and genetics. Indeed, scientists have identified a gene that is implicated in some forms of Alzheimer's.

Does that mean Alzheimer's can be detected with a genetic test?

Not quite. In 1993, a link was discovered between a form of the gene ApoE, called ApoE4, and increased chances of getting Alzheimer's disease. Since then, a great deal of research has been done, and a lot of arguing has been going on. ApoE4 is specifically associated with two types of Alzheimer's disease, sporadic and late-onset familial. What's important to remember, however, is that the test only indicates an increased risk. There are many people with the gene who never develop Alzheimer's and many without the gene who do. Research is moving quickly, but as of this writing, it is estimated that between 23 and 57% of people who actually have Alzheimer's disease would be misdiagnosed if this gene were the sole criterion for the diagnosis.

Does the gene ApoE4 cause AD?

Let us reiterate that no one actually *knows* what causes AD. To quote a thoroughly researched and comprehensive article by T.D. Bird, M.D., of the University of Washington Medical School, "Although impressive strides have been made in the past decade elucidating the molecular mechanisms underlying AD, the precise pathogenesis of the disease remains unclear." However, some scientists believe that the defective gene causes an ineffective synthesis of cell membranes in the brain. Then the immune system, which is not always our friend, attacks the faulty cell membranes by overproducing an immune system messenger called interleukin-6. This stimulates a brain chemical called beta amyloid to break off from its parent molecule, amyloid precursor protein (APP). In the final step, beta amyloid causes free-radical damage to brain cells, resulting in neuron death in the area of the brain that is responsible for producing acetylcholine. Because acetylcholine is crucial for memory and cognition, its deficiency causes the symptoms we recognize as Alzheimer's.

What are the symptoms of AD?

Basically, the symptoms include memory problems and loss of intellectual abilities that are, in the words of the Alzheimer's Association, "severe enough to interfere with routine work or social activities."

Which of the types of memory we discussed before is affected by Alzheimer's disease?

Primarily, it is the short-term, episodic memory that goes first. In other words, a person with Alzheimer's may remember in detail his or her own history—stories about her first prom, reminiscences about his wedding, the names of college roommates. S/he may still be able to recite poems memorized in childhood and reel off the names of the states in alphabetical order. What will be affected first is the ability to remember whether s/he has already put the salt in the soup and the bread in the oven. The severity of the problem, of course, is a matter of judgment. Forgetting an occasional phone number or having trouble remembering a name is not a cause for concern. That can happen to a healthy 16-year-old. Because the onset of Alzheimer's is gradual, however, more serious symptoms may be noted even before they form enough of a pattern for certainty.

How can you tell when you should be concerned?

The following quiz, adapted from a checklist compiled by the Department of Health and Human Services, may help clarify this issue. Use the questions to help you evaluate the condition of the person you are concerned about.

- Does s/he have trouble learning and remembering new information, such as recent conversations, events, and appointments?
- Is s/he becoming more repetitive? Does s/he tell you the same thing three or four times?
- Has s/he started to have trouble with complex tasks that s/he used to be able to handle, such as balancing a checkbook or cooking a complete meal?
- Does s/he seem stymied by a problem s/he would once have been able to respond to, such as a flooded bathroom or a broken flowerpot?

- Does s/he have trouble driving, organizing objects around the house, or finding his or her way around a familiar place?
- Does s/he have more and more difficulty finding the right words to express what s/he thinks or feels?
- Does s/he have trouble following conversations?
- Is s/he becoming more passive, less responsive to people and situations?
- Is s/he increasingly irritable and/or suspicious?
- Does s/he often misinterpret what s/he sees or hears?

If you must answer "yes" to any number of these questions about the behavior of a family member or friend, there is sufficient cause to suggest a talk with his or her doctor or psychologist. The doctor can then get a better idea of the situation in a number of ways. The simplest is probably trying to engage the patient in conversations about an area in which s/he knows the patient has an interest. The doctor can also look for other changes in behavior over a number of visits. Once the doctor decides that there is evidence of dementia, s/he must determine whether the cause of it is Alzheimer's or some other, possibly reversible, condition.

What is dementia?

Although there is some disagreement about the exact meaning of this word, we are going to use it to refer to the impaired mental performance that results from some physical condition, such as Alzheimer's. It is not itself a disease. Rather, it is a group of symptoms that can result from any of a number of different diseases and physical conditions. A relatively small percentage of all older people are afflicted by dementia caused by Alzheimer's disease or a related condition, but the problem is one that increases greatly with age. The latest research in the field indicates that 1% of the population age 65 to 74 has severe dementia. That proportion increases, however, to 7% of those age 75 to 84 and 25 to 45% of those 85 or older. Still, it is imperative to remember that this is not a normal part of aging but the outcome of a specific disease, injury, medication, or other contributing cause. In any diagnosis of Alzheimer's, it is crucially important to eliminate as possibilities these other causes.

What are some of these other causes of dementia?

There are a number of them. When we do an examination, we hope to find causes that are reversible. They include things as widely varied as depression, head injuries, brain tumors, systemic disorders such as infections, toxins, drug side effects, metabolic disorders, and nutritional disorders. Often, an older person who appears to be developing Alzheimer's is actually suffering from the loss of interest in the outside world that accompanies depression. S/he is not incapable of remembering. S/he just doesn't care anymore. This

condition can be treated with talk therapy, antidepressant drugs, or a combination of the two.
Other patients are already taking various prescription drugs and may be losing brain function as a
side effect. More than once, taking a patient off a
drug has produced a miraculous "recovery" from
what was thought to be encroaching Alzheimer's.
In other cases, it may be discovered that a patient
is neglecting his or her diet to the extent that serious nutritional deficiencies have resulted. A return to a balanced diet, and perhaps supplements,
can do the trick.

Are there other irreversible causes of dementia, besides AD?

Unfortunately, there are quite a few. They include
vascular disease, repeated strokes or mini-strokes,
Pick's disease, Creutzfeldt-Jakob disease, Parkinson's disease, and AIDS. Pick's and Creutzfeldt-
Jakob diseases are rare, and our knowledge of
them is very limited. Pick's affects fewer than
three-tenths of one percent of the population and
is characterized by literal shrinkage of the brain. It
can usually be identified with a CAT scan.
Creutzfeldt-Jakob is even rarer, affecting no more
than about 300 people in the United States at any
given time. It is caused by a virus, and most patients die within a year or so of diagnosis. Again,
brain changes can be identified with a scan.
Parkinson's disease is a disorder of the central nervous system that becomes more severe as the disease inevitably progesses. In later stages of the disease, dementia can appear. All three of these

diseases can cause a deterioration of intellectual faculties in the sufferer, as can the final stages of AIDS.

Isn't there any way to diagnose Alzheimer's with a blood test or some such thing?

Unfortunately, there is not at this time a single diagnostic test for Alzheimer's. When symptoms appear that cause concern, your physician can do a complete physical and run tests that may rule out other possible causes for the symptoms. The examination should include the following:

- A complete health history, including a review of any medications being used
- A physical examination
- Blood tests to rule out disorders involving kidneys, thyroid, and liver, as well as tuberculosis, pellagra, and pernicious anemia
- A questionnaire concerning mental status
- A neuropsychological examination which tests sensory and motor functions.

Other tests which may be performed include the following:

- EKG (electrocardiogram) to measure heart arrhythmias and enlargement of the heart
- PET (positron-emission tomography) to scan the brain for changes, abnormal blood flow, and metabolic disturbances
- EEG (electroencephalogram) to examine brain waves

- CT (computerized tomography) to rule out
  the presence of blood clots or any evidence
  of stroke
- MRI (magnetic resonance imaging) to provide an overall picture of the brain.

According to the Alzheimer's Association,
when this kind of examination is done on a patient, a physician's resultant diagnosis of Alzheimer's is about 90% correct. One hundred percent certainty comes only after death and an
autopsy of the brain showing neurofibrillary tangles and neuritic plaques.

What about testing for the ApoE4 gene? Couldn't that tell people they have Alzheimer's even before they get symptoms?

Genetic testing is always tricky, but in this case it
can be downright misleading. The first thing to
remember is that about 65% of those with AD do
not have an ApoE4 gene, so a negative result
would not rule out the disease. In addition, the
test is not currently recommended for young
people who have not shown the symptoms. Such
an individual who tested positively would have
only about a 30% chance of developing AD. For
older people who have shown signs of dementia,
as we have pointed out, a clinical diagnosis is correct about 90% of the time. Adding testing for
ApoE4 can increase that percentage to 97, but the
two should go together. The ApoE4 test alone is
not at all conclusive.

Can Alzheimer's be cured?

No. At the present time, there is no cure for Alzheimer's. Research continues all the time, but so far scientists have been unable to find anything that can cure or reverse the destruction caused by the disease. That's why the early studies on ginkgo are so promising. As we will explain, the LeBars study in the JAMA actually showed *improvement* in the mental abilities of the patients who were given ginkgo biloba.

Can Alzheimer's be treated?

In the past few years, two drugs have been put on the market that can make some impact on the symptoms of the disease. Tacrine (brand-named Cognex) and donepezil (brand-named Aricept) are both cholinesterase inhibitors. People with Alzheimer's have a deficiency of the neurotransmitter acetylcholine, for some reason. There is another chemical in the brain, the cholinesterase enzyme, which gobbles up this crucial neurotransmitter. These two drugs prevent that gobbling process. Unfortunately, tacrine is not terribly effective and has the dangerous side effect of liver damage. Donepezil works somewhat better and does not affect the liver. It does, however, cause stomach upset, which can be mitigated somewhat by taking the drug at bedtime. But neither of these substances is a miracle drug. So far, there is not a really good treatment for the disease. A number of other substances are now being studied. They include vitamin E, estrogen, non-

steroidal anti-inflammatory agents, and ginkgo
biloba.

What does ginkgo biloba do for Alzheimer's sufferers?

Apparently, ginkgo helps patients perform better
mentally and may even repair some of the damage
that has already been incurred.

What is the evidence for this improvement?

Let's begin with the breakthrough study by
LeBars and his colleagues, as it was published in
the *Journal of the American Medical Society*. The researchers recruited 309 people with dementia believed to be caused by Alzheimer's and vascular
disease. Half of the subjects were given the ginkgo
biloba extract EGb 761—40 mg. three times a
day—and the other half were given a placebo.
Neither subjects nor researchers knew who got
what. The patients were given a battery of tests
for mental functioning, particularly with regard to
short-term memory. The tests were given at the
beginning of the study, before the patients began
taking the ginkgo. They were then repeated at 12
weeks, at 6 months, and at the end of the yearlong
study. At the 6-month point, the results of one
particular cognitive test were striking. On this
test, Alzheimer's patients are expected to lose four
points in 6 months. Instead, 27% of those taking
ginkgo showed a four-point improvement. It
should be pointed out that 14% of those taking
the placebo showed a similar improvement, prob-

ably because of the attention being paid to all the patients. Still, it was an important indicator and one worth paying attention to.

Then, at the end of the trial, the ginkgo group scored better on two of the three important tests than the placebo group did. On the third test, there was no difference. In addition, improvement was reported by the ginkgo patients' caregivers. The authors of the study stated that "EGb 761 was safe and appears capable of stabilizing and, in a substantial number of cases, improving the cognitive performance and the social functioning of demented patients for 6 months to 1 year." Although this is not a definitive study, it's difficult not to be excited about the potential of a substance that could actually *improve* the mental abilities of patients with Alzheimer's. The study clearly points the way for further research.

Is this the first study to show that ginkgo helps people with Alzheimer's?

By no means. A review in the British *Journal of Clinical Pharmacology*, as far back as 1992, looked at 40 studies that investigated using ginkgo extract for "cerebral insufficiency." The review eliminated 32 of those studies as failing to meet strict scientific standards, but the remaining 8 studies all showed that patients taking ginkgo showed significant improvement. In a recent edition of *Prevention* magazine, writer Mark Bricklin cited a number of studies, including one by the German Association of General Practitioners. In their inquiry, which involved 209 patients, 71% of the ginkgo patients showed an improvement over 12 weeks, as opposed to 32% of the placebo group. (There's that attention factor again.) Another study, reported in *Human Psychopharmacology* in 1994, gave a battery of tests to 40 subjects, then gave half of them 240 mg. a day of EGb 761. After 1 month, there was significant improvement on all tests, and that improvement continued for the 3 months of the study.

A review of existing studies, which was published in a French medical journal as far back as 1986, came to this conclusion: "the drug [ginkgo biloba extract] seems to be effective in patients with vascular disorders, in all types of dementia, and even in patients suffering from cognitive disorders secondary to depression, because of its beneficial effects on mood. Of special concern are people who are just beginning to experience deterioration in their cognitive functions. Ginkgo biloba extract might delay deterioration and enable these subjects to maintain a normal life and escape institutionalization."

These are only a few of the studies that have been done in Europe, over the past few decades, on the various properties of ginkgo. What's different about the study published in JAMA is that it was done in the United States, it was carried out over a fairly long time, and it used standardized testing instruments to measure the intellectual improvement, or lack thereof, in its subjects. In other ways as well, it met the highest scientific standards.

Then what do its critics say is wrong with it?

There are a number of points being raised by those who believe that too much attention is being paid to the study. They point out that only 202 of the original 309 patients finished the year-long trial. They wonder why there was no improvement on the third test for cognition that was given to the subjects. They say that the difference between the ginkgo group and the placebo group was not great enough to bear the weight of the study's conclusions. However, the most important criticism is that the media and the public are putting altogether too much importance on what is, after all, a small, early study.

This criticism, if you can call it that, is true. And the authors of the study agree. Because of the media attention given to the study, its significance has been blown out of proportion. However, this study did show that there is real *potential* in the herb ginkgo, and there are even now larger and longer-term studies being carried out. In addition, ginkgo has a history. It did not appear overnight, just as this study was begun. As physicians and informed consumers, we can look at other indicators, including the status of the herb in Eastern medicine and in Europe. Given the remarkable safety of ginkgo, we have some latitude in making our evaluations, and these factors can weigh in our decisions.

How does ginkgo work to help Alzheimer's patients?

There are a number of different theories about that. What's interesting is that all three of ginkgo's known properties might be involved. It is an anti-inflammatory and an antioxidant and it increases blood circulation, as we pointed out before. Any of these properties, or any combination of them, might affect dementia.

How could an anti-inflammatory drug help Alzheimer's patients? Would any anti-inflammatory drug—such as aspirin—help?

It's not clear yet how, but research has indicated that people who take anti-inflammatory drugs are one-tenth as likely to get Alzheimer's as those who don't. That's a very impressive reduction in risk. The reason this is true has not yet been determined. Indeed, we don't know for sure that there is a causal relationship. However, the fact is there. It was discovered when scientists at the National Institute on Aging (NIA) and Johns Hopkins University carried out a 15-year study, using data from NIA's Baltimore Longitudinal Study of Aging, and published the results in the March 1997 issue of *Neurology*. This was not a controlled study but rather an examination of data generated by the NIA. The Johns Hopkins scientists found that anti-inflammatory drugs such as ibuprofen, taken for as little as 2 years, appeared to reduce the risk of Alzheimer's disease. Acetaminophen, which has no anti-inflammatory properties, had no effect on the incidence of Alzheimer's. Oddly, aspirin, a potent anti-inflammatory agent, also appeared to have little or no effect on the risk of Alzheimer's within the parameters of this study. Researchers speculate that the amounts taken were too small.

The study was conducted by Walter F. Stewart, Ph.D., at Johns Hopkins School of Public Health; Claudia Kawas, M.D., and Maria Corrada at Johns Hopkins School of Medicine; and E. Jeffrey Metter, M.D., at the NIA. Kawas stated, "Many scientists now believe that inflammation may be an important component of the Alzheimer's disease process. The amyloid and protein plaques found in Alzheimer's patients' brains, which are hallmarks of the disease, may be indicative of an inflammatory response."

Obviously, given the study's negative experience with at least one anti-inflammatory drug—aspirin—it is difficult to make a firm statement about the possibilities of ginkgo without direct research. But it is clear that the anti-inflammatory properties of the herb *may* be involved in the improvement it makes in memory. And because frequent, long-term use of most anti-inflammatory drugs can lead to serious side effects, including peptic ulcers and impaired kidney function, it would behoove scientists to include ginkgo in any further studies on Alzheimer's.

What about the antioxidant properties?

LeBars and his colleagues on the study reported in JAMA believe that this is where the answer lies.

They state: "The mechanism of action of EGb [761] in the central nervous system is only partially understood, but the main effects seem to be related to its antioxidant properties. . . ." What antioxidants do is scavenge for free radicals, which have been implicated in some of the damage observed in the brain of an Alzheimer's patient. Ginkgo, in other words, gets the free radicals before they can get the nerve cells. LeBars and his colleagues go on to point out that these properties depend on the extract as a whole, rather than just the ginkgolides, for example, or the bioflavonoids.

You said all three of the important properties of ginkgo could be involved. What about the third one?

The third property of ginkgo that could be involved is its ability to increase blood circulation. This is the most attractive, commonsense explanation, as well as the one that is most appealing to people who hope ginkgo can sharpen undamaged memories. Oxygen is necessary to the functioning of the brain, the reasoning goes. Blood carries oxygen to the brain. Ginkgo helps get *more* blood to the brain. Therefore, ginkgo makes the brain function better. This line of reasoning is almost certainly true, but it is important to remember one word—"enough." If a brain has "enough" oxygen, is ginkgo going to help by bringing it more? Maybe and maybe not. But that's a question for another chapter.

Could all three of these properties be working together in the Alzheimer's patients?

Absolutely. Indeed, it seems very likely.

Could ginkgo help prevent AD?

It seems to us that research should now be directed toward answering that question. Here is a safe, relatively inexpensive herb that has been shown to have some effect on people whose condition is already far enough advanced to be diagnosed. What might it do to prevent the condition from ever making its appearance? If the free-radical theory is true, prevention—at least to some degree—seems to be a real possibility. At any rate, the research community certainly should address this.

Would you recommend combining ginkgo with any other treatments?

Yes. To begin with, if you are a postmenopausal woman, you might consider taking estrogen.

Is estrogen considered a treatment for Alzheimer's?

In a sense, that could be one of its properties. In every current survey of research into Alzheimer's, estrogen is mentioned. It is being considered as a way of preserving the cognitive capabilities of women after menopause. As we mentioned in the

Alzheimer's chapter, women are at greater risk for the disease than men are, and the risk increases with age. It now appears that one of the advantages of hormone replacement therapy for women might be to lessen that risk. Recently, researchers from Johns Hopkins reported on a study of 472 women over a period of 16 years. About 45% of the women had, at one time or another, taken estrogen. The estrogen users, according to the study, were 56% less likely to develop Alzheimer's than those who had never used it.

The mechanism involved, according to current theory, is that estrogen makes the nerve cells more sensitive to the hormone NGF (new growth factor). It also stimulates the production of acetylcholine! That, you remember, is the crucial neurotransmitter that is deficient in Alzheimer's patients and that is involved in memory. In that sense, estrogen would be a memory enhancer. That does not mean, of course, that it would have the same effect on young women . . . or men.

The potential of estrogen as a factor in mental fitness is so great that the National Institutes of Health (NIH) has begun a study on estrogen and Alzheimer's at 38 medical centers in this country. The subjects of the study will be 8,000 healthy women who are 65 years old or older and who are already taking estrogen.

Is there anything you would recommend for both men and women?

Considerable research has gone into nondrug therapies for Alzheimer's, and we would strongly recommend that these be practiced. They include the following:

- Work with your physician to monitor any possible symptoms.
- Keep yourself in the best physical condition you can. This includes as much activity as you are physically capable of—and can fit comfortably into your life—as well as balanced nutrition.
- Take care of your emotional health, combating anxiety and depression with talk therapy and/or antidepressant medication.
- Undergo memory training. This training is most effective when undertaken with a group, either using a manual or with an instructor.
- Increase your intake of antioxidants (ginkgo; vitamins A, C, and E; and especially glutathione and lipoic acid).

There are also a number of other supplements you might want to consider, including coenzyme Q_{10}, the B vitamins, and DHA (docosahexaenoic acid), which are dealt with in some detail in Chapter 7.

These are simply guidelines. You should also consult your own physician about what s/he recommends.

Chapter 3

Ginkgo, Memory, and Normal Aging

The research is accumulating to show that ginkgo biloba can help repair and maintain memory in people with Alzheimer's disease. Is the same true for other people, perhaps those who are experiencing the normal processes of aging? Probably the first thing we need to look at—to answer this question—is the process of memory itself.

Memory is crucial to the efficient working of all aspects of human reason, and it is at the emotional center of our lives. (How many songs have been written about deductive reasoning?) It is also the focus of most of our efforts for mental improvement because it is the aspect of cognition that is most obvious and disturbing in its absence. And yet, our understanding of memory—what it is, how it works, why it fails—is often vague and incomplete. Before we can look at the options available for enhancing this crucial aspect of our intelligence, we need to know what we are dealing with.

What is memory?

Probably the simplest way to put it is that memory is the brain's record of what we experienced in the past, whether that is an instant ago or a decade ago. Remembering is retrieving that record, bringing it back into the conscious mind.

Sort of like pulling it out of a filing cabinet?

That's a comparison that's used a lot. It's a nice, simple analogy with considerable appeal. It has only one real problem. It is almost completely misleading. The magnitude of the operation is so different from anything a computer is capable of that the difference becomes one not just of size, but of kind.

When the director of the Brain Research Institute at UCLA was interviewed by *Fortune* magazine in 1990, there was a black-and-white photograph of the Andromeda galaxy on his desk. That galaxy contains about 100 billion stars, which is approximately equal to the number of cells in one human brain. Furthermore, each one of those nerve cells, or neurons, in the brain can maintain a *million* communication links with other neurons. So, each human brain has the capacity for one million times one billion connections. *Fortune* explained the implications of that this way. "If a computer were built to replicate the brain's network, it would occupy a ten-story building covering the entire state of Texas." That's Texas, you understand, not downtown Manhattan or even Rhode Island. One brain. Of course, computer technology has advanced enormously since 1990.

It's possible that we would now be able to knock off a few of those stories. Still, it's an impressive image.

Obviously, pulling one memory out of *that* filing cabinet requires more than a good knowledge of the alphabet. And yet, somehow, each one of us does it all the time. The least sophisticated person in the world plucks out bits of data about events of a dozen years ago with such ease that he or she never even wonders how. *We* are going to wonder how, though, because understanding how the process works will make it easier to understand how it fails and what we can do about it.

How do things get into the filing cabinet to begin with? How do we acquire memory?

That happens constantly. Everything we see, hear, or feel—everything we taste, smell, or think—becomes, for at least an instant, the subject of a memory. Some of those memories stay with us forever, while others are lost as soon as our brain decides, for whatever reason, that they are not important. And even those may not really be wiped out, but simply lost to our retrieval system. In a sense, the memories we keep for ready reference are of things we have "learned."

You mean, like reading or riding a bicycle?

Well, yes, but the term "learning" can be misleading. It suggests a complex process, and although many of our memories are complex, others are as simple as the smell of bacon. Perhaps

a better way of putting it is to say that we remember things that have "made an impression"
on us, however slight.

Where do memories go in the brain?

We're not really sure. And when we talk about
memories, we have to use images that could be
misleading.

When we talk about "storing" and "retrieving"
memories, about where a memory is located and
how we find it, we are using a metaphor, not an
exact description of what happens in the brain.
For all our sophisticated technology and the advances made possible in neuropsychology, we
don't *know* exactly what happens in the brain. We
just know a lot more than we used to.

All right, where are memories kept in the brain?

Apparently, memories are located in certain of the
neurons in the brain, perhaps in the part of the
neuron called the axon, which is dedicated to
communication with other cells.

One neuron contains one memory?

Not exactly. Memories are not isolated. There appear to be memory chains, called *memory traces*,
linked by a flow of electric current. The neurons
in the memory traces don't actually touch each
other. They are separated by tiny gaps that are
called synapses. A thought, as we understand it,

must flow from one cell to another by means of chemicals called neurotransmitters. Six out of the approximately 100 neurotransmitters in the body seem to be assigned the responsibility for brain function, and the one most crucial for memory appears to be the neurotransmitter called acetylcholine.

No one is absolutely sure how memory traces are created, but it is now established that a memory may be stored in more than one part of the brain at once. Therefore, communication between different parts of the brain must remain open and fluid if our memories are to function properly. This means that we must have not only abundant neurotransmitters but also intact, functioning neurons.

How do we store memories?

In roughly three different ways. *Sensory register* is the almost instantaneous registering of a sensory stimulation. *Short-term memory* occurs when we log something for a few seconds or perhaps days, just for immediate use, and then "forget" it. *Long-term memory* is the fairly permanent acquisition of data.

What is an example of sensory register?

Let's say that you're cooking. You take a pot off the stove and your mind registers that the burner is still on. You turn it off and continue with the preparation of your meal. You have no particular reason to remember this commonplace event—

unless you're about to leave the house—and so you don't.

What is an example of short-term memory?

The classic example is that you look up a phone number in the directory and, without writing it down, you dial the number. If you get a busy signal and then try to dial the number again, you'll probably have a good reminder of how short "short-term" memory can be.

What is an example of long-term memory?

Your name. How to ride a bicycle. The capitals of the states (if you ever learned them). Your wedding anniversary.

Does this help explain why I can remember the name of my third-grade teacher and not what I was supposed to pick up at the store?

Exactly. Short-term memory passes into long-term memory by the process we referred to earlier as "learning." If you haven't learned something, you won't be able to remember it for long. You apparently "learned" the name of your third-grade teacher well.

But then, why can amnesiacs, who can't even remember who they are, remember how to ride a bicycle? Aren't those both long-term memories?

Yes, they are. But there are, as it happens, two different kinds of long-term memory.

What are they?

One is called *procedural*, and it involves "remembering how." That's where bicycle riding comes in—along with walking, talking, reading, and thousands of other things that we learn how to do as we go through our lives. Usually, this kind of memory is a result of practice, or repetition. It is very durable. *Declarative* memory, on the other hand, involves "remembering that." People who are very good at this win large sums of money on *Jeopardy*. It includes remembering the names of things, for example, and the categories into which they fall. "That object is called a saw and it is a tool." Declarative memory is considerably more fragile than procedural memory.

What is the most fragile sort of memory?

Probably a form of short-term, declarative memory called *episodic memory*. It involves remembering events from your own life, such as looking into the cabinet before you go to the store and seeing that there is no cereal. This seems to be a problem in retrieving information, not in acquiring or storing it. You saw the space on the shelf where the cereal was supposed to be and recorded that fact, but you were unable to bring it to the surface of your mind when you got to the store.

How do we retrieve (or use) memory?

If you've ever worked with a computer database, you know that you can index one entry in many different ways. Take the following as an example:

Jane Doe, performance artist
Innovative Theater Company
1234 Little Broadway Boulevard
Hollywood, Idaho

You can program your database to retrieve Jane when you type in any of the following parameters: artists, performers, theater members, performance artists, Idaho artists, Western artists, Hollywood performers, people named Jane, people named Doe, etc. That sort of indexing and cross-referencing has become enormously sophisticated, even on your home PC. What the most advanced computers can do is truly staggering.

However, the human mind somehow cross-references hundreds of thousands of aspects of one simple visual memory, so that you can retrieve the image of a particular tree, for example, when you see a certain color of green, hear a sound like the rustle of leaves, or touch a roughness like bark; and also when you think of Jack, who stood beside you as you looked at the tree; or when you hear the name Aberdeen, which was the town near the forest. It can even happen when you bite into a salami sandwich, which reminds you that you couldn't find salami one day and had to settle for bologna, which is how you found out that Jack loved bologna, which he insisted on taking on every picnic thereafter, except for the one you took to that forest near Aberdeen, where you ate a lunch of chicken salad near a lovely lake under a tall alder tree. Bingo.

What about people who can remember whole bridge games or chess games? Do they have a special kind of retrieval system?

Not really. We all do that. It would be a staggering feat if they were remembering unconnected items. However, if you think of the entire game as one memory, a kind of picture inside the brain, it becomes less dumbfounding. The expert consults that picture, all the parts of which fit together in a way that makes sense to him or her, in order to find each individual bit of information. This sort of "picture" is a crucial aspect of the way human memory works. When you are asked, "What color hair does your Aunt Jane have?" your memory probably presents you with a "picture" of your Aunt Jane that includes her hair color, rather than sorting through zillions of unrelated bits of hair-color information in the hair-color storeroom of your brain.

So, when we talk about enhancing memory, are we talking about enhancing the *acquisition* of memory, the *storage* of memory, or the *retrieval* of memory?

That is an extremely important question, because people may mean different things at different times. Some may be looking for a way to improve the learning process, which involves the acquisition and storage of memory, while others are seeking a way to eliminate "absent-mindedness," which probably involves the retrieval process.

Which kind does ginkgo biloba work on?

Some of the studies of ginkgo biloba have involved taking large doses immediately before studying written material or attempting to master a procedure. Those studies are testing the effect of ginkgo on the learning process, the acquisition and storage of memory. Other studies, such as the Alzheimer's study, have addressed the retrieval of memory. The most promising aspect of ginkgo, *according to tests done so far*, is with the retrieval of short-term, episodic memory—the kind that helps you remember what to get at the grocery store. However, there are indications that it can help with different kinds of memory *in certain people*.

Clearly, a substance that is effective in one situation may or may not be effective in another. As we look at ginkgo and other memory enhancers, keep that in mind. If you want to improve your short-term, episodic memory—which is the goal for most of us—you should deal skeptically with claims based on tests involving learning, such as memorization or maze-running. It's important that you—as a reader, patient, and consumer—focus on the type of memory you want to improve so that you can make an intelligent decision about your options.

Who are the people ginkgo is most likely to help, besides Alzheimer's sufferers?

Probably people who are no longer in their youth. Most of us suffer some memory loss as we get older, and there is a strong possibility that ginkgo can be of use in that case. The fundamental issue that remains unresolved is whether memory deterioration is a necessary part of the aging process or whether the memory loss that usually occurs after the age of about 40 is a result of controllable factors in our bodies and our lives. To determine that, we have to look at the brain itself and how it ages.

What does happen to the brain as it ages?

The best way to explain this is to start with what happens to the brain at the beginning of life. This is something that new technology is only now beginning to reveal to us. Using something called positron-emission tomography (PET), pediatric neurobiologists can now "watch" the activity in various sections of an infant's brain in a noninvasive procedure. What they have discovered is that the brain's 100 billion neurons have formed more than 50 trillion connections at birth. This "basic wiring," as writer Sharon Begley put it in a 1997 *Newsweek* article, is dictated by the baby's genes. It makes certain that the baby's heart will beat and its lungs breathe. Amazingly, that's about all it does. In the first months of life, the brain will make *20 times* that original 50 trillion connections. One thousand trillion is a lot of connections, and even the body's 80,000 different genes couldn't possible make them all. They are made primarily by the baby's experience with the world. The more stimulation a baby has—in the form of games such as "peekaboo" and "this little piggy"—the more connections are made.

Does all this connection forming take place at the same time?

No. What is happening during this time is actually the structuring of the mind, physiologically as well as psychologically, and it takes place in stages. This process is called *synaptogenesis* and it involves the formation of synapses, those tiny gaps between neurons that we discussed earlier. At right around 2 months, it begins in the motor cortex. That's when babies lose their "startle" and "rooting" reflexes and begin to perform purposeful movements. At about 3 months, synaptogenesis reaches its peak in the visual cortex. You will see the baby begin to focus its eyes on specific objects. It isn't until about 8 or 9 months that synaptogenesis begins to complete itself in the hippocampus, which is where memory lives.

Does that mean we start remembering when we are 8 or 9 months old?

Yes, in a sense. As 9-month-old infants, we can remember, for example, that if we squeeze a rubber toy it will make a noise. We can make the kind of mental connection that allows us to master simple learning processes. This is not to say that we form long-term memories that we will be able to retrieve when we are in our twenties. There are those who say we do, that the memories are there somewhere and the problem lies in our ability to retrieve. Someday we will probably know the truth about it, but now we can only say that infants are forming memories of some kind in the second half of their first year. At the same time, the prefrontal cortex, which is the home of logic and forethought, starts forming synapses at an astounding rate. For the next 10 years of the child's life, that synaptogenesis will, according to Begley, consume *twice as much energy as an adult brain.* Considering that the adult brain uses 20% of the body's energy (while taking up only about 3% of its bulk), that's an impressive amount of energy and one reason that good nutrition is so important in a child's mental development.

When does all this brain structuring stop?

That's the amazing thing. It doesn't. We used to think that it did, but we now know that, although it comes to a sort of natural end during adolescence, it can be restarted. All those billions of neurons get assigned tasks early on, but it is possible for the brain to *reassign* tasks if necessary, as in the case of damage to one part of the brain. The brain, while fragile (those neurons are not capable of reproducing themselves), also seems to be remarkably adaptable.

Still, most of each brain's structure is determined in the first decade or so of life. The brain learns what life is like and adapts itself to deal with what it finds. If life, for a particular child, is marked by danger and uncertainty, the brain learns to produce the chemicals that keep us wary and alert to danger. If life is regular, dependable, and filled with comfort and safety, the brain becomes better at producing the chemicals that allow us to remain calm and anxiety-free. That is a bit of an oversimplification, of course, but in essence that's the way the process seems to work.

How is memory affected by a child's negative experience?

It has been discovered that, in adults who were abused as children, the hippocampus is smaller than in other adults. The hippocampus, remember, is the seat of memory. Scientists believe this is the result of stress hormones washing through the brain. Clearly, the reverse is true of children who are cherished and nurtured.

How does memory functioning change as we grow up and grow old?

Although there is controversy surrounding this subject—as there is with any aspect of cognition and/or aging at the moment—there is a useful distinction to make here. Human intellect may be seen as having two aspects: *crystallized intelligence* and *fluid intelligence*. Crystallized intelligence involves the skills we learn through education and practice. Reading, for example, is a "crystallized" skill. Fluid intelligence includes nonverbal reasoning, motor skills, and problem-solving abilities that change and evolve as the individual matures physically. Coping with a flooded bathroom is, no pun intended, a "fluid" skill.

Now, an excellent article in the *Western Journal of Medicine*, entitled "Memory, Thinking, and Aging: What We Know about What We Know," explains that "crystallized abilities—such as knowledge of general facts and vocabulary—sharply increase during the early years of formal education and then stabilize or gradually improve throughout adulthood." For most of us, this rings true in terms of our own experience. We learn an enormous amount of life-changing information in grade school and continue to learn, although less rapidly, all through our lives. Watching a program on the Discovery channel when we are in our fifties, we learn that eagles and timber wolves have been taken off the endangered-species list and we add it to whatever general knowledge we may have about wildlife. And we remember it. A pundit being interviewed on a talk show uses the word "intransigent," and we look it up or ask someone what it means. And it becomes part of our vocabulary.

On the other hand, according to Sharon Begley in her 1997 *Newsweek* article, "fluid abilities improve throughout childhood, then gradually decline in adult years, with more deterioration in old age due to neuronal loss, changes in physiologic brain function, and increased rates of disease and injury." This too has a commonsense appeal when we realize that this category includes reaction time, speed of perception, and the ability to focus and concentrate. We may get wiser as we get older, but we seldom get sharper.

So we get a little fuzzier as we go along, but when does real deterioration of memory and other thinking skills start?

This is where we really get into controversy. Many psychologists and physicians consider memory loss in people over 40 to be a clinically definable, *physiological* condition. This "condition" is called Age-Associated Memory Impairment (AAMI) or Age Related Cognitive Disorder (ARCD). AAMI is recognized by the National Institutes of Health. Dr. Thomas Crook, at the Memory Assessment Clinic of Bethesda, Maryland, has been working for several decades to analyze memory and age. He and his team have worked out a number of tests that are designed to measure and evaluate memory decline in age. According to Robert Smith, in an article in *Total Health*, these tests are "objective and precise, yet they are savvy and built around common everyday tasks like grocery shopping, driving, reading, meeting a stranger and later having to match the face with the name, and so on." Crook has tested people, in both the United States and Europe, chosen at random and grouped by age. Their studies confirm that there is a decade-by-decade decline in cognitive abilities. In the appendix to this book, several tests of the kind used by Crook and other researchers are included, with age-related scoring. You might be interested in testing yourself.

Does this decline in memory happen to *everybody*?

That's the big question, of course. Crook and his followers believe that it does. They define ARCD as a non-disease, age-related decline. The National Institutes of Health also believes that there is a physically determined change in memory. There are many arguments in favor of this view. However, there is an opposing view that is quite plausible and gaining currency in the medical community. Many medical professionals and cognitive researchers believe that there is no preordained deterioration of the molecular and cellular mechanisms of memory. They insist that any damage to the brain is caused by factors other than age.

What are the factors that these scientists believe are damaging our brains?

To a great degree, they are the factors in our life and environment that cause free-radical damage. In her book *Stop Aging Now!*, health-writer Jean Carper writes, "Many prominent investigators now view aging not as an inevitable consequence of time, but as a disease itself—the ultimate conglomerate disease caused by a lifetime of environmental assaults to cells . . . . Aging occurs when cells are permanently damaged by continual attacks from chemical particles called free radicals. Simply, the cellular damage accumulates over the years, until the totality of destruction reaches the point of no return—diseases clustered at the end of life and eventually death." In other words, "age" is not a matter of time, but of free-radical damage.

Is the brain particularly vulnerable to free-radical damage?

Yes, it is, for a couple of reasons. To begin with, free radicals are the product of a process called oxidation. It's very much the same process that makes apples turn brown or butter become rancid. As we explained before, a free radical is an oxygen molecule which has lost one of its electrons. Because the brain uses 20% of the body's oxygen intake, it's often exposed to possible damage. Second, neurons are unable to reproduce themselves; therefore, dead and damaged brain cells are not replaced. They are gone forever. And though it's normal to lose a certain number of brain cells gradually, over time, no one can afford to lose more than they have to.

What are some of the causes of free-radical damage, and therefore memory loss, in the brain?

In his enlightening article "No Way to Treat the Mind," Steven Rose cites a recent Dutch study from the University of Limberg, Maastricht, which reports that "memory decline in otherwise healthy people as they age is associated with mild head injury, general anaesthesia, or 'social drinking' earlier in life."

Smith makes a similar point and cites Dr. Robert Sapolsky, a researcher at Stanford University. Sapolsky points out that other causes of mental deterioration include sustained emotional stress, glutamate (as in monosodium glutamate), smoking, pollutant substances, and lifestyle drugs (both legal and illegal). All of this is consistent with free-radical damage.

So, memory loss may be due not to age itself, but to the free-radical damage that accumulates as we get older?

That's one theory, and it's an important one. But in some ways it's like saying that wrinkles are not caused by age but by sun. That's true, but to most of us it doesn't make any difference. We have been exposed to the sun all our lives. We will continue to be exposed to it for the rest of our lives, and we have wrinkles as we get older. Period. As for the causes of memory loss, most of us have had experience with one or all of the three contributing factors mentioned in the Dutch study. Presumably "mild head injury" includes whacking your head on the sidewalk when you fall off your bike at the age of 12. Certainly most of us had general anaesthesia when we had our tonsils out, and some of us have had to undergo surgery in later life. Social drinking, of course, is very widespread in this culture. As for Sapolsky's list, most of us, of course, have been exposed to a number of these in our lifetimes. Therefore, even if you don't accept age as a clinical condition causing mental deterioration, it is probably safe to say that most people—

by the age of 40—could use a little help in the memory department.

Life may begin at 40, but do good memories end there?

We said a *little* help. Unless you have Alzheimer's disease or some other specific form of what is called dementia, you probably won't notice any serious changes until you're over 70. And even then your verbal abilities and other crystallized intelligence should remain unchanged.

The largest study of aging and cognitive changes is being carried out in Seattle. It is called the Seattle Longitudinal Study (SLS) and has been observing more than 3,000 mentally healthy adults since 1956. Each subject is given a battery of tests every 7 years in five areas: verbal meaning, spatial orientation, inductive reasoning, number skills, and word fluency. So far, the SLS has discovered that performance in all these areas begins to decline by about the age of 74. However, most participants in the study keep or increase their level of performance in at least one area. In other words, if you are particularly good at Scrabble, you will probably still be able to beat your teenaged nephew when you're in your seventies, *even* if you're not as quick as he is at figuring out how to put together a set of prefabricated shelves.

What do these thinking skills have to do with memory?

Memory is involved in all cognition. Think about it. Without memory, you would not be able to put one word after another. You have to remember the first word in order to add the second. Without memory, you would not be able to add two plus two or keep a thought in your mind long enough to come to a conclusion. It might be too much to say that thought is memory, but it's close.

What if I don't want to resign myself to this gradual memory loss?

The most obvious answer is to take antioxidants to combat free-radical damage. Ginkgo biloba is an important one. The LeBars researchers theorize that it was the antioxidant properties of ginkgo that produced positive results in the study of Alzheimer's patients. Ginkgo is a potent, safe source of antioxidants.

What other sources of antioxidants are there?

There are a number of others. Plants and the food we derive from plants are the major sources of these valuable substances. Indeed, fruits and vegetables are the first line of defense against free-radical damage.

To begin with, plant foods provide the antioxidant vitamins E, A, and C. In addition, there are other antioxidants available in specific foods. For example, tomatoes contain the antioxidant lycopene, soy-protein foods contain isoflavones, red wine contains polyphenols, broccoli contains sulphoraphane, and strawberries contain ellagic acid. Green and black teas also contain polyphenols in large amounts. Five cups of tea supplies the same quantity of antioxidants as two servings of fruit or vegetables. When trying to obtain antioxidants from food, go for what is freshest and protect the nutrients in your food until you can get them into your body.

Are there any antioxidant supplements I can take?

Many neuroscientists recommend vitamin E supplements. Daily doses of 2,000 IU, in at least one study, improved the ability of early Alzheimer's patients to cook, dress, and eat, and it was quite probably the antioxidant properties of the vitamin that caused the improvement.

Could ginkgo counteract "normal" memory loss in any other way?

Quite possibly. To explore its potential, we could do worse than to look at the factors that researchers have discovered in older people with good mental fitness.

What *are* the factors that contribute to mental fitness as we age?

For just over a decade, the MacArthur Foundation Network on Successful Aging has been sponsoring research into this question. Fifteen scientists around the country have been carrying out studies into factors as varied as genetics, psychology, environment, and sociology. In one study, almost 1,200 healthy adults between the ages of 70 and 80 were tested for 22 different variables. The tests took place in 1981 and then again in 1988. What the director of the study—Marilyn Albert, Ph.D., of Harvard University Medical School—discovered were four crucial factors. They were the following:

- Level of education
- Level of physical activity
- Lung function
- Feelings of self-efficacy.

Two of these four factors directly involve increasing the amount of oxygen that reaches the brain. Both physical activity and good lung function contribute to feeding the brain the oxygen it needs. So, too, does ginkgo. What's more, because of its vasodilator properties, ginkgo can help bodies that are no longer young keep up their level of physical activity.

So you're not suggesting that I take ginkgo *instead* of exercising?

Absolutely not. And we're not suggesting that you take ginkgo instead of continuing your education, formal or otherwise. An interesting article in *Psychology Today*, entitled "Making Our Minds Last a Lifetime," quotes memory researcher James L. McGaugh, "There's growing neurobiological evidence that supports the commonsense notion of 'use it or lose it.' The brain may be more like a muscle than we ever thought."

Decades of experience with physical-fitness fads and foibles has taught us that the best way to get a strong, fit body is to exercise it. The same appears to be true of the mind. Other contributing factors such as nutrition are important, but they cannot make up for a mind that is allowed to get flabby with underuse. Taking ginkgo will almost certainly help you keep your mind in good trim. Reading books that challenge you to think and push your skills of comprehension a little harder than you're used to will probably help just as much.

Chapter 4

Ginkgo and Other
Memory Problems

On the basis of studies done with Alzheimer's patients, many young, healthy people are buying ginkgo biloba to enhance their own memories. They are making a great leap from the available data to the desirable conclusion. Is that leap justifiable? We can look at some other information about ginkgo biloba to help us decide.

Can ginkgo biloba help memory in young people?

That's certainly the claim being made. Television ads call it "the thinking person's supplement." It's always listed with the herbal and nutritional equivalents of "smart drugs," along with ginseng, choline, and the like. There is a great deal of anecdotal evidence that suggests it can help memory in some people, evidence that it would be narrow-minded to ignore.

However—and this is a big however—it probably can't help everyone. There's only one way to find out whether it is likely to help you, and that is to look at the individual properties of the herb and relate them to specific forms of memory loss with specific causes.

Could ginkgo's ability to increase blood circulation help memory in young people?

Possibly. Even critics of the current wave of interest in ginkgo admit that the herb can make it possible for more blood, and therefore more oxygen, to make it to the brain. What the critics are quick to point out, however, is that more oxygen may not do you any good unless you begin with a *deficiency* of oxygen in the first place. Varro Tyler, Ph.D., professor emeritus at the Purdue University School of Pharmacy and author of *The Honest Herbalist*, puts it this way, "The group for which studies have shown that ginkgo improves short-term memory and concentration consists of people with impaired blood flow to the brain." Since circulation problems increase with age, probably most people from their forties on experience less than perfect blood flow to all parts of the body. Most studies of ginkgo and memory show the greatest benefit to people in this age range. However, aging is not the only cause of deficiency in this area. Older people are not the only ones with impaired blood flow to the brain.

Who else might have a deficiency of oxygen?

We can begin with a population that has traditionally been given ginkgo in China—asthmatics.

There has been a tremendous increase in asthma in this country among all ages, and though we could not find specific studies concerning ginkgo and cognition in asthma sufferers, it would seem to be a profitable area for research. The same would seem true for sufferers from other respiratory problems, such as allergies.

What about the antioxidant effect? Could that help younger brains?

That is an important question. After all, LeBars and his colleagues believe that it is the antioxidant properties of ginkgo that were involved in the improvement of cognitive functioning in the Alzheimer's study. As we explained before, free radicals of oxygen are created in the body during the normal processes of life but are also created by disease, injury, smoking, and air pollution. They bombard healthy cells, causing damage that we believe may induce skin aging, cancers, and aging of the brain. Antioxidants combat these free radicals.

Damage from free radicals is cumulative, becoming more serious as we get older. Therefore, it stands to reason that the antioxidant properties of ginkgo would have a greater effect on older people. Again, ginkgo would benefit older rather than younger people, but younger people who have had significant free-radical damage may be exceptions. More studies need to be done here, but it makes sense that a young woman of 26 who has been smoking since she was 15 may benefit from a strong antioxidant.

Does that mean young, healthy people can't benefit from using ginkgo?

In this society at this point in history, 40 is considered young—if not medically, then culturally. Ask Cal Ripken. Not to mention Cybill Shepherd. So, if we accept that there are physical changes affecting cognition that begin as early as 40, then we must say that ginkgo may very well be able to help "young, healthy people."

What about people younger than 40? Can college students and young businesspeople use ginkgo to get a "competitive edge"?

Jamison Starbuck, a licensed naturopathic and homeopathic physician who uses ginkgo extensively in her practice, says that she awaits further studies on ginkgo and young minds. However, she states, "I can offer this observatory note: since I practice family medicine in a university town, I frequently treat student-patients seeking natural medicines that will help them with difficult midterms and finals. While both young and old have tried ginkgo, I have noticed that it is the older students who seem to most benefit from taking ginkgo. Is this the result of maturity, better study habits, or the age-appropriate use of ginkgo biloba? Time, perhaps, will tell."

Starbuck's reservations are echoed by most researchers and physicians. Ginkgo just doesn't seem to have the impact on *most* young people that it does on *most* older people. That's one point.

But there's another point here, of equal importance. In addition to age, we need to look at the kind of memory aid these young people are looking for. Is it the kind that ginkgo can provide?

What kind of memory can ginkgo enhance?

So far, the evidence indicates that ginkgo helps short-term, episodic memory, the kind that is most problematic for Alzheimer's sufferers. It may very well help other types of memory, but there is no real proof of that yet. If what you're looking for is something to help your *learning* ability, ginkgo is almost an unknown factor. There is one frequently cited study that was published in the *International Journal of Clinical Pharmacology*, in 1984, in which 12 healthy young women were each given 600 mg. of ginkgo extract 1 hour before performing memorization tests. They were reported to have performed better than when they didn't take ginkgo. However, that study has not been duplicated. Indeed, when it was tried with a different group of 12 young women, there was no improvement. And those initial results have not been confirmed in the 15 years since then. What's more, 600 mg. is a very large dose. The recommended daily dose is about 120 mg.

This is not to say that ginkgo *can't* help you learn, just that we don't yet have evidence that it can. We do have evidence that it can help people, especially older people, stay on top of their everyday lives.

Are there *any* young people ginkgo could help with their short-term memory, just as it does older people? Is age really what's at issue here?

As we've explained, impaired blood flow to the brain and free-radical damage can result from other causes besides age. One possibility is a serious deficiency of certain important nutrients. Some researchers have tended to ignore this fact, assuming that most Americans are reasonably well nourished.

Well, aren't we? Aside from people who live in desperate poverty, most Americans don't actually suffer from malnutrition, do they?

"Malnutrition" suggests something quite extreme to most of us, so let's not use that particular word. Instead, let's simply talk about serious deficiencies of important nutrients. According to James G. Penland, a research psychologist at the U.S. Department of Agriculture's Human Nutrition Research Center in Grand Forks, North Dakota, a great many Americans suffer nutritional deficiencies as a result of dieting (in the case of women) or (in the case of men) from consuming foods too high in fats and too low in vitamins and minerals. Unfortunately, such deficiencies are particularly prevalent among "young" women. The incidence of bulimia among female colleges students in this country is startlingly high. A deficiency of only one vitamin, B_{12}, can lead to irreversible memory loss and other neurological problems, if it persists for long enough. This is not to say that bulimic college students should count on ginkgo to pass their exams. In all of these cases, the first step is to correct the nutritional imbalance. However, ginkgo may be an additional aid.

Is there any other portion of the young population who might want to consider ginkgo?

There are a great many young people who have spent their entire lives exposed to pollution in all its forms, and the incidence of asthma is soaring in this country, probably as a result of environmental factors. In Eastern medicine, the treatment of asthma is one of the major uses of ginkgo. In addition to the breathing benefits asthma sufferers may receive, ginkgo should also benefit their cognition as the result of improved oxygen flow to the brain. It certainly seems that this is an area researchers could profitably look into. In the meantime, because ginkgo is such a safe herb, people of any age who have respiratory difficulties—and do not take blood thinners—might consider taking ginkgo.

I have Chronic Fatigue Syndrome (CFS), and it seems to cause problems with memory and concentration. Could ginkgo help that?

That's one of the areas currently being researched. There are no completed studies that we know of, but there are indicators that ginkgo could be useful for both CFS and Fibromyalgia.

Given the safety of ginkgo and the limited number of options that exist for the sufferers of these two debilitating conditions, a self-trial could very well be indicated.

So, young people may be able to benefit from ginkgo?

In some cases, yes. There may be numbers of young, apparently healthy people who have suffered damage to the nerve cells or who have problems with circulation. Those people might benefit from ginkgo. This is not to say that bulimic college students should count on ginkgo to pass their exams. Or that ginkgo is a substitute for better regulations concerning air and water pollution. It is far better to go to the root of the matter and address the nutritional deficiency or other cause. When that is not possible, however, ginkgo may be able to help.

What needs to be done to determine how effective ginkgo is as an aid to memory in people who have no organic problems?

Large studies of younger people need to be conducted, using standardized measurement instruments, such as memory tests that have been used and proved in other contexts. These studies need to be long-term enough to test, not just the blood-flow enhancement, but the corrective effects of ginkgo's antioxidant properties. In other words, researchers should not be taking 12 college students and giving them 600 mg. of ginkgo an hour before giving them a test. A conclusive study would take several hundred people, using placebos in a double-blind situation. It would involve taking a reasonable dosage of ginkgo for at least 12 weeks, preferably longer. Results from such a study would give us some real confidence in the use of ginkgo by people under 40 who have no discernible organic problems.

Could it hurt to take ginkgo now, before more tests are run?

Almost certainly not. Virtually everyone agrees, whether critical of its effectiveness or not, that ginkgo biloba is safe. Even the notoriously conservative Food and Drug Administration (FDA) classifies the herb as "probably safe." The one important exception, as we mentioned before, is that one of the properties that makes it useful for increasing blood circulation could be dangerous to people who are already taking blood thinners because of heart problems. There have also been rare difficulties for people with low blood pressure.

In a recent article in *Natural Health* magazine, 12 experts in the field of cognitive health were asked what supplements they took themselves. These experts ranged from a research neuroscientist at Harvard Medical School to a practitioner of Chinese medicine to the author of a popular book on smart drugs. Two of these experts took no supplements of any kind. Of the remaining 10, half took ginkgo, more than any other single supplement.

In effect, you can run your own subjective test of ginkgo. What you should keep in mind if you are going to try the herb are the following:

- Take 120 mg. each day. Most preparations come in 40-mg. dosages, but that is only one-third of the amount used in most clinical studies, including the LeBars study on Alzheimer's.
- Take ginkgo for at least 12 weeks. A shorter period of time will not give you a clear picture of what is happening.
- Talk to your doctor about what you are doing. If you expect resistance, be prepared to explain your decision. Some people like to write down things that they are afraid they will forget to mention in their doctor's examining room. One of the appendices to this book is a fact sheet you can fill out and take to your doctor to help you explain why you would like to try ginkgo.

After this test, you should have some sense of whether ginkgo is helping you or not. If you can't tell, ask people who are close to you whether they have noticed any difference. If they can't tell either, it's probably safe to say that you are not a good candidate. Yet.

Chapter 5

Other Uses of Ginkgo Biloba

Although the focus of this book is ginkgo biloba as a memory enhancer, it is impossible to make a study of this remarkable herb without noticing its many other uses. A great deal of research has been done, with results that are often striking. When you are making your decision about ginkgo, some of these additional benefits may tip the balance for you. We can begin with some of the ways ginkgo might be able to improve the functioning of your senses.

What senses does ginkgo benefit?

It has been shown to benefit vision and hearing, as well as the "sense" of orientation, which includes our equilibrium, or balance.

How does ginkgo benefit vision?

There are a number of factors that contribute to good vision. Of course, heredity plays a big part.

If your genes say that you are going to have to wear glasses, you will. However, taking care of the eye itself will determine whether you have the best vision it is possible for you to have. As you know, the eye has to adjust to see objects at different distances. As you get older, its ability to adjust lessens. A child with normal vision, for example, can see clearly objects that are as close as 2½ inches from the face. By 30, the average person has trouble with anything closer than 6 inches. And at 60, most of us cannot see clearly anything that is closer than 16 inches.

German scientists in the early 1990s did a study on 25 people in their seventies, giving some of them EGb 761 at a dosage of 160 mg. a day and some of them the same extract at 80 mg. Within 4 weeks, those on the higher dosage began to show improvement in their vision. The scientists reported that these subjects showed a "significant increase in retinal sensitivity," as measured by a new system to study the health of the retina. When those on the lower dosage were given 160 mg., they too showed improvement. Of significance is the fact that the more damaged retinas showed the most improvement. Two other studies on animals, rather than humans, showed similar results. One took place at the Institut Henri Beaufort in France and the other at the University of Leipzig.

Why did ginkgo help to repair the retinas of these subjects?

There are probably two reasons. To begin with, the tissues of the retina are rich in fatty acids, which are particularly vulnerable to free radicals. For that reason, the antioxidant properties of ginkgo would be very helpful in protecting and, it seems, repairing the retina. Second, the retina requires a great deal of fuel. That fuel, in the form of oxygen and glucose, may be helped to get to the eye by the blood-circulation properties of the herb. These same properties may be involved in the benefits ginkgo seems to have for people with age-related color-blindness.

Can ginkgo actually cure color-blindness?

It appears to be useful in age-related color-blindness. Color vision seems to peak in the thirties and decline thereafter. For most people, this is not a particularly serious problem. We still distinguish color as well as we need to for everyday life and for the appreciation of the beauty around us. For some, however, this reduction in the ability to see and distinguish colors is severe. Georges M. Halpern, Professor Emeritus of Medicine at the University of California-Davis, points out that the great artist Georgia O'Keeffe was afflicted with this form of color-blindness in her later years. And there is at least one study that showed improvement in the ability to distinguish colors after 6 months of taking ginkgo. That study was done in the late 1980s in France on 29 subjects. However, there is not yet a body of evidence to confirm these findings.

Can ginkgo help the eye in any other way?

There is a possibility that it can help to slow the development of macular degeneration. We need to be cautious about making this claim because the degeneration of the macula, which is part of the retina, is a truly heartrending condition, and raising false hopes is not what this book is about. However, there was one study done in France, and reported in September 1986 in *La Presse Medicale*, that indicated ginkgo may be of use for sufferers from this condition.

Macular degeneration is a condition suffered by many in old age. When it begins, the insulation between the retina and the blood vessels behind the retina starts to break down, with the result that fluid leaks into the retina. Scar tissue begins to form. This scar tissue builds up in the center of the macula, causing a blind spot in the center of the visual field. Gradually, the spot grows, and the victim's visual ability is reduced. Reading becomes impossible. Then driving becomes out of the question. While the peripheral vision endures, the individual can usually get around in familiar environments, and then that ability diminishes.

The French study was carried out on 10 subjects with macular degeneration. Half were given ginkgo and half a placebo. The conclusion of the study was that those given ginkgo had an improvement in their distance vision. Although this study is not even close to conclusive, it indicates an important area for research. And it suggests another reason—to those of us who are past 40 and beginning to think about the ravages of aging—for adding ginkgo to our daily regime.

In what ways can ginkgo biloba help the sense of hearing?

There is evidence that ginkgo can be useful in cases of damage to the cochlea, which is the snail-shaped passage at the front of the inner ear. The cochlea contains the sensor receptors for hearing and is vulnerable to damage from a number of sources. Exposure to loud noise is one cause of acute cochlear deafness. So, too, is infection. Damage to the cochlea is also a side effect of certain drugs.

In 1986, a French study was done on patients who were in the early stages of acute cochlear deafness. Half were given ginkgo and half were given an alpha blocker. Fifty-two percent of those taking ginkgo showed substantial improvement in their hearing, while 35% of those taking the alpha blocker showed improvement. Another study was done the same year on 20 subjects whose deafness was caused by a sudden event, such as an explosion of sound or a loss of pressure in an airplane cabin. Again ginkgo and alpha blockers were compared, and again ginkgo significantly outperformed the drug.

The researchers in these studies concluded that ginkgo's ability to increase circulation was one of the reasons that it was effective in these cases of cochlear damage. They also noted that, according to Halpern, "it protected cells and blood vessels in some unspecified way." Twelve years later, we can speculate that the protection may stem from ginkgo's antioxidant properties.

Can ginkgo do anything for chronic deafness?

So far as we know, there is absolutely no evidence that ginkgo can benefit those who suffer from any form of deafness other than acute cochlear deafness.

I have tinnitus. I've heard conflicting reports about ginkgo's ability to work on this condition. Does it really work?

There are very good reasons for the mixed messages you're receiving. One reason is the very nature of the disorder. Because tinnitus is a ringing, roaring, or hissing sound perceived as "inside the ears" by those who suffer it, there is no objective way to measure the severity of the condition or any improvement in it. This excerpt from an Internet discussion on ginkgo and tinnitus is very revealing:

1. I saw my ENT [Ear, Nose, and Throat specialist] yesterday for a 6-month checkup. I have Ménière's & T. [tinnitus]. I asked him about Ginkgo, as I began taking it about 5 weeks ago. He said not to bother; it hasn't

been proven to help unless perhaps a placebo effect. But, he said it doesn't hurt a person. He said people grasp for anything they think might help. I guess I'll finish the second bottle I bought & see how I am then. Good luck. Vicki

2. If the medical profession haven't got the foggiest idea as to how T. is caused or what to do about it, it seems a bit naive and arrogant for your ENT to say what does or for that matter does not work. I find that Ginkgo not only helps (and I have tested this—time and again—by stopping and starting again) but also reduces the volume of the T. substantially for me. It is not a cure but an effective "volume-control" for me. Ian

3. Mr. Hinds may be "lucky" in that his tinnitus is caused by restricted blood flow. For that case, ginkgo biloba can help as it specifically improves blood circulation. For all other cases, ginkgo biloba does nothing. Don't believe in false hope. Earthling

4. Well—the absolute certainty expressed, especially in the statement that Ginkgo "does nothing," is impressive.

And so it goes, for pages. Most of the tinnitus sufferers reporting had tried ginkgo. Most of those thought it helped. A few said it was no help at all. Research studies have also had contradictory results. In one study of patients who had been referred to the Department of Audiology at Sahlgren's Hospital in Göteborg, Sweden, the results were as ambiguous as it is possible to get. Out of 20 patients, 7 preferred ginkgo to the placebo, while 7 preferred the placebo to ginkgo, and 6 had no preference. The study concluded that "since there is no objective method to measure the symptoms, the search for an effective drug can only be made on an individual basis."

The Swedish scientists also pointed out that tinnitus has several different causes. It is possible that, as "Earthling" stated, ginkgo is primarily helpful to those whose ringing is caused by circulatory insufficiency. There is at least enough evidence for any tinnitus sufferer to try the herb for him or herself.

If ginkgo can help problems in the ear, can it help with equilibrium problems, like vertigo?

There is a very good chance it can. Both German and French studies have had positive results in this area. A German study done recently at the Medical University of Lubeck investigated the effect of ginkgo on patients with vertigo and nystagmus (involuntary eye-rolling), the result of damage caused by temporary stoppages of blood to different parts of the brain. The 36 patients in the study were between 45 and 73 years of age. Eighteen of the patients were given ginkgo in the form of EGb 761 and 18 were given a placebo. The patients were required to perform standardized exercises and balance-training once a day, and their eye movements were investigated both clinically and by means of a machine designed to measure such movements.

Interestingly, ginkgo did not help the nystagmus, but it did have a significant effect on the vertigo. "The intensity of vertigo decreased significantly more in the EGb 761 group [by 46%] than in the placebo group [by 14%]," according to the researchers.

This study confirmed findings of a 1986 study by French researchers on 67 patients who had suffered from balance problems for less than 3 months. Thirty-four of the patients were given 160 mg. of ginkgo each day; the rest were given a placebo. Using a variety of measurements and standard tests, the researchers determined that, after 90 days, 74.7% of the subjects taking ginkgo had improved, as opposed to 18.3% of the placebo group.

What other conditions can be helped by ginkgo biloba?

Let's begin with the conditions that are most closely related to those we have been discussing. Varro Tyler, in *The Honest Herbalist*, writes " . . . there is an impressive body of literature attesting to the effectiveness of Ginkgo Biloba Extract (GBE) in treating ailments associated with decreased cerebral blood flow, particularly in geriatric patients. These conditions include short-term memory loss, headache, tinnitus, depression, and the like." The benefit in these cases is not limited to geriatric patients, and ginkgo is also useful for conditions involving decreased blood flow to other parts of the body. Ginkgo has long been used to aid circulation, and recent studies have verified its efficacy in this area. The conditions that have been shown to benefit from ginkgo's cardiovascular properties include peripheral arterial insufficiency, vertigo, tinnitus, vascular headache, intermittent claudication, diabetic tissue damage, and circulatory disorders of the skin.

How can ginkgo help my thrombosis?

Thrombosis is the formation of a blood clot within a blood vessel. It is a painful and dangerous disorder. In clinical studies, ginkgo reduced the tendency for thrombus formation in veins and arteries. It also lowered blood pressure and dilated peripheral blood vessels in patients recovering from thrombosis. These results suggest many possibilities for the herb's use in the prevention and treatment of coronary thrombosis and in the recovery from strokes and heart attacks. In one 1992 study, German scientists treated 20 patients with 240 mg. of the standardized ginkgo extract for 12 weeks. The nonhospitalized patients suffered from a coronary heart disease, hypertension, high cholesterol levels, and/or diabetes. At the end of that time, the substances in the blood that promote clotting had decreased in every single patient.

Obviously, this is an area where self-medication is far too dangerous to contemplate. However, it might be useful to ask your physician to consider ginkgo in this situation.

I have pains in my legs, and my doctor says that's because I have bad circulation. Can ginkgo help me with this?

Very probably it can. "Bad circulation" is a simple name for disorder of the peripheral arteries. Several clinical studies have shown that people with peripheral arterial disease can walk for significantly longer periods of time without pain after taking ginkgo. In one German journal article in 1992, all known "placebo-controlled, randomized and double-blind studies with the major target objective of pain-free walking distance" using either EGb 761 or a drug called pentoxifylline, already accepted as a treatment for this disorder, were summarized and evaluated. The conclusion of the article was that the increase in walking distance was highly variable from patient to patient, especially in the pentoxifylline studies. However, on average, ginkgo produced an increase of 45%. The drug results were somewhat higher, at 52%. Given that ginkgo is safe and relatively inexpensive, this seems to make it a good option.

This is the sort of study that confirms what traditional use of the herb suggests. Its results make sense in terms of what we already know about ginkgo's ability to enhance blood circulation. The combination of folk wisdom, common sense, and science is an excellent basis for making a decision about what you are willing to try for yourself.

What conditions might be helped by ginkgo's anti-inflammatory properties?

The most important one, traditionally, is asthma. Asthma, as we pointed out earlier, is overreaction on the part of the respiratory system to relatively harmless irritants. When they sense an "attack" by irritants, they go on the defensive, becoming inflamed. Since the lungs are not being damaged by the trigger but by the inflammation, modern asthma therapy involves using steroids to reduce the inflammation that shuts off air passages and causes asthma sufferers to gasp for air.

Ginkgo biloba, as a potent anti-inflammatory, could be very useful for mild cases of asthma or for patients who cannot or do not want to use steroids. If you fall into one of those categories, talk to your doctor about giving ginkgo a trial run. *Do not, under any circumstances, change your asthma therapy without talking to your doctor.*

Could ginkgo help with arthritis?

It makes sense that it would, if you're talking about osteoarthritis. Anti-inflammatories have long been used to treat arthritis. In addition, a July 1997 article, in *Annals of the Rheumatic Diseases*, reports on several studies that have found a connection between the use of antioxidants and improvement in osteoarthritis. The author of the report, Timothy McAlindon, M.D., suggests that antioxidants may not only slow the progress of arthritis; they may also actually repair damage. They do not, however, prevent arthritis, acting only after the damage has occurred.

Given the efficacy of both anti-inflammatories and antioxidants, it would make sense that ginkgo could help. However, we have not found studies that support this commonsense conclusion.

What other possible benefits are being investigated?

Studies are being done on dozens of conditions, including diabetic retinopathy, diabetic tissue damage, arteritis, cerebral edema, arterial blockage, and even hair regrowth.

Isn't this all a little too good to be true? After all, can an herb really be a "wonder drug?"

Let us reiterate that not all these studies have been successfully concluded or confirmed. Many are in the initial stages of research. At the same time, it is important to remember that ginkgo has three potent properties. And each of these properties has many, many applications. A list of the conditions that benefit from the use of any anti-inflammatory, for example, would be quite long. Add to that the conditions that could benefit from the use of an antioxidant and an aid to blood circulation and you get an impressive list indeed.

Ginkgo biloba may not be a wonder drug, or herb as the case may be, but it is certainly a powerful substance that is ready to move from the herbalist's notebook to the physician's desk reference.

Chapter 6

Ginkgo, Sex, and the Reproductive System

Sexuality is at the center of human life, and problems that arise in connection with it are among the most difficult and emotionally painful we can experience. For some time, it has been clear to those in the health and medical fields that overall good health is a crucial factor in the proper functioning of the reproductive systems in both men and women. As gingko contributes to your gaining and maintaining a high level of general health, it will as a matter of course improve your sexual and reproductive health. However, there are also specific ways in which gingko can be of use in this area of life.

Can ginkgo do anything for my PMS?

The answer to that seems to be a resounding yes. Given the pain that premenstrual syndrome (PMS) causes in the lives of its sufferers, and the problems that medicine has encountered in trying to treat it, that is very good news.

91

PMS is a condition that afflicts most women . . .
to one degree or another. That last qualifier is a
terribly important one. The majority of women
are uncomfortable, physically and/or psychologically, for a day or two a month. A tiny minority of
women suffer from severe symptoms that include
clinical depression, constant breast pain, and even
suicidal impulses. Obviously, there's a huge range
between these two extremes. However, all PMS
sufferers have one thing in common. They hate
the medical establishment. For as long as anyone
can remember, doctors have been telling women
that their hormonally related symptoms were all
in their minds. Even after PMS was brought out
into the open, in the last few decades, doctors
continued to refer their patients to psychiatrists
with a nonchalance that was staggering. In fact,
two researchers in Chicago announced in 1998
that they were launching a study to find out
whether PMS exists.

There have probably always been negative as-
sociations with menstruation and the premenstrual interval. However, the recognition of a
cluster of symptoms regularly occurring before
the menses came only in 1931, by an American
gynecologist named Dr. T. Frank. About 80% of
all women experience some premenstrual symptoms. Somewhere in the neighborhood of 2 to 5%
experience PMS as a serious interruption to their
daily functioning.

How is PMS diagnosed?

Doctor and patient keep track of symptoms for 2
or 3 months. The symptoms that are considered

in the diagnosis are those that occur only in the 7 to 10 days before menstruation. Any symptom that also occurs the rest of the time is not considered a sign of PMS. These symptoms include the following:

Group A
- A depressed mood, feelings of hopelessness
- Anxiety and tension
- Sudden and dramatic mood swings
- Anger and irritability

Group B
- Decreased interest in usual activities
- Difficulty in concentrating
- Fatigue, lack of energy
- Change of appetite, overeating, food cravings
- Sleep disturbances
- Sense of being overwhelmed
- Physical symptoms such as breast tenderness or swelling, headaches, joint or muscle aches, bloating, weight gain.

In order to make a diagnosis of PMS, the doctor would look for five of these symptoms, with at least one in the first group.

Aren't there treatments and medications for PMS sufferers already?

There are some. For many years, it was thought that PMS might be caused by a deficiency of progesterone, one of the two important "female" hormones. As a result, the condition was treated with supplementary progesterone. More recently it has been suggested, however, that PMS is *actually* caused by estrogen, the balancing hormone for progesterone. In the last several years, the medication of choice for PMS has been Prozac or one of the other selective serotonin re-uptake inhibitors (SSRI). These have been very helpful with the depression and anxiety that are often part of PMS—and with food cravings. They are, however, more than many women want or need to deal with their symptoms, and they do not address the pain and water retention that can make PMS so uncomfortable.

Can ginkgo help with the pain and water retention of PMS?

Yes. A French study was done just a few years ago on 165 women, between the ages of 18 and 45, who had "congestive premenstrual troubles" during at least 7 days of their cycle. It was a double-blind study in which half of the women received gingko and half a placebo. Before any medication was given, 1 month was spent evaluating each woman's symptoms. Then, symptoms were rated for the 2 months during which the medication was taken. Both the patient herself and her practitioner rated the symptoms. At the end of the study, scientists concluded that gingko was effective against congestive symptoms, especially breast swelling and tenderness.

Does ginkgo do anything for the anxiety and depression of PMS?

Yes. The conclusion of the French study also stated, "Neuropsychological symptoms were also improved." In other words, patients felt less anxious and depressed. This could easily have been the result of reducing water retention and breast pain. It might, on the other hand, have something to do with the anti-inflammatory effect on tissues, or even with gingko's effect on the brain. There is no way of telling, in such a subjective test. There were no side effects reported, and the gingko did not affect the women's hormonal balance.

Since there are so few effective therapies for severe PMS, it seems that giving gingko a trial period of 3 months would be quite a reasonable decision. This should be especially effective if the PMS patient is already observing, or begins to observe, other guidelines for the disorder, including the following:

- Avoid caffeine. This is difficult, but it is also the single most effective step that medical science has discovered for the treatment of PMS.
- Reduce your sodium intake. This should help with edema.
- Increase your intake of potassium-rich food such as bananas, yogurt, kiwi fruit, potatoes, and cantaloupe. This, too, helps with water retention.

- Eat carbohydrates. This increases your serotonin level, which helps both mood and
  sleep disorders.
- Exercise often. This may be as important as
  avoiding caffeine.

On a regimen of this kind, with the addition of
gingko, it might be possible to avoid more extreme measures, such as antidepressant or anti-
anxiety medication.

Does ginkgo have any effect on male impotence?

It can, depending on the cause of the condition.
Impotence is not in itself a disease. It is a
symptom of some underlying problem, psychological or physiological. Ginkgo seems to be
useful with impotence that has certain physiological causes.

What are the physiological causes of impotence?

Impotence, of course, is the inability to achieve
and sustain an erection. An erection, however, is
not a single act. It is a process that involves nerve
impulses in the brain, spinal column, and genital
area as well as responses to those impulses in the
muscles, veins, arteries, and fibrous tissues in that
area. The most common cause of impotence is
damage to the arteries, smooth muscles, and fibrous tissues. About 70% of all cases of impotence
involve damage caused by diseases, including dia-

betes, kidney disease, chronic alcoholism, multiple sclerosis, atherosclerosis, and vascular disease. Between 35 and 50% of all men who suffer from diabetes experience impotence. In addition, surgery can cause damage that results in impotence, as can other kinds of injury.

Unfortunately, impotence can also be caused by many common medicines, including high-blood-pressure drugs, antihistamines, antidepressants, tranquilizers, appetite suppressants, and cimetidine (an ulcer drug). Smoking, which affects blood flow in veins and arteries, may cause or contribute to impotence. And insufficient testosterone can also be a cause.

Isn't a lot of impotence psychological?

Actually, no. Psychological factors are believed to *contribute* to impotence in situations where there is a physiological basis. But most experts in the field believe that psychology causes long-term impotence in only about 10 to 20% of cases.

What kind of impotence can gingko help?

One study has been done with gingko and men who suffered impotence as a side effect of taking SSRIs (selective serotonin re-uptake inhibitors) such as Prozac and Paxil, as well as other antidepressants. Alan Cohen, a psychiatrist and professor at the University of California at San Francisco, carried out an open trial of various oral formulations and found ginkgo effective in 84% of patients with sexual dysfunction caused by antidepressants. He first discovered the potential of gingko when one of his elderly patients asked if he could try it for his memory. Cohen had tried treating the man's sexual dysfunction—a side effect of antidepressants—with a number of other substances, to no avail. A month after beginning to take gingko daily for his mind, the man reported a great improvement in his ability to obtain and keep an erection. (His memory was also doing better.)

When the trial began, the first six patients receiving the herb responded positively to it. "Seeing a 100% response," Cohen stated, "I proceeded to use gingko on an ongoing open-enrollment basis. After 2 years, more than 100 patients have enrolled in the study. Five of the six original patients are still using gingko, and all types and classes of antidepressant have been used. One patient was on an MAO inhibitor and did not suffer any adverse reaction." The side effects recorded by Cohen were all mild and could usually be relieved by gradually reducing the dosage until the body could tolerate it. These side effects included various kinds of gastrointestinal upset. Cohen's patients begin with a dosage of 120 mg. per day. This dosage is slowly increased to 480 mg. per day, in two doses. Dr. Cohen has recently received grant approval for a formal, double-blind study of gingko and SSRI-related sexual dysfunction.

Can ginkgo help in any other form of impotence?

There is evidence that it can, especially in cases where the problem is poor circulation in the arteries of the penis. A 1989 *Journal of Urology* article reported on a study in which 60 men who suffered from this form of impotence were given 60 mg. of gingko daily for 12 to 18 months. At the end of the study, half of the men were able to have erections. In a 1991 study, 50 men were given a daily dose of 240 mg. of gingko. Some of the men in the study had previously benefitted from drugs in treating their impotence and some had not. Those who had reacted positively to drug treatment also reacted positively to gingko. All of them. Those who had not reacted positively to drugs experienced improved circulation in the penile arteries but did not report real success in achieving erections.

Clearly, more research needs to be done in this area. However, if you are a man who experiences impotence as a side effect of antidepressants or because of circulatory problems, it would seem that trying gingko is indicated.

Chapter 7

Other Natural
Memory Enhancers

If ginkgo biloba does not seem to address your particular concerns with regard to memory, there are a number of other options you might want to consider. Some of them, like ginkgo, have been around for ages. Others are only now being added to the arsenal of weapons against cognitive degeneration and simple forgetfulness. Quite a number of them have come out of the search for a cure for Alzheimer's. At the moment, Alzheimer's research is the most important memory research being done. The danger associated with this is that we will know only about drugs and other herbs that are effective on damaged brains. They will not always be drugs that can help healthy brains.

What are the options available to me to enhance my memory?

Basically, they fall into four categories. There are herbs, such as ginkgo and ginseng. There are the supplements that duplicate substances the body produces itself, such as DHA, PS, ALC, and DMAE. There are basic nutrients, including vitamins and minerals, as well as omega-3 fatty acids, and amino acids. Then there are also some recently developed "smart drugs," such as piracetam and Hydergine.

Which herbs are believed to enhance memory?

There are a number of herbs, especially from Chinese and Asian medicine. One of the oldest, and in some ways the most important is the herb many people confuse with ginkgo—ginseng.

What is ginseng?

Ginseng is the common name for the Araliaceae, a family of tropical herbs, shrubs, and trees grown in Asia and North America. The use of its root in medicine goes back at least 2,000 years, to China's Han Dynasty. It is most frequently described as a "tonic," or adaptogen, a medication that improves overall stamina and performance. In addition, say its proponents, it protects the liver, calms nerves, normalizes the cardiovascular system, and prolongs life. Given so many claims for its powers, it may come as no surprise that the genus name of the Asian variety, *Panax ginseng*, reflects the Greek word panacea, a medicine for all ills. There is an American variety called *Panax quinquefolius*, which was discovered in 1716 in Canada and has since been exported to China. Siberian ginseng is not a real ginseng. Its botanical name is *Eleutherococcus senticosus*.

What is the active ingredient in ginseng?

That would be the ginsenosides. More than 20 ginsenosides have been extracted from different types of ginseng. Siberian "ginseng" does not contain ginsenosides. However, both the Panax forms and Siberian ginseng are mild stimulants of the adrenal nervous system and the cholinergic nervous system.

Why do you consider ginseng so important?

Ginseng is one of the most widely used medicinal substances in the world. Until the recent boom in the popularity of ginkgo biloba, it was the most popular herb in the United States. A lot of people believe in it and a lot of people use it. Like ginkgo, it has thousands of years of folk wisdom behind it. *Unlike* ginkgo, however, it has never been endorsed, however mildly, by JAMA.

Have any studies been done into the effectiveness of ginseng?

In China, Japan, and Korea, there have been many studies. Subhuti Dharmananda, director of the Institute of Traditional Medicine, a nonprofit group in Portland, Oregon, says, "They claim good results, but if you show them to researchers in the United States, they will throw them in a round filing cabinet." There have been more conventional studies as well. At a 1974 International Ginseng Symposium, Swedish researchers reported that college students who took Panax ginseng every day had better test scores than a control group and reported improved concentration. What's interesting about this study, done in 1974, is that it is still being cited in articles about ginseng. Does that mean that there have been no better, more recent studies?

In other countries, such as Russia, Siberian ginseng has been tested on older patients, with some evidence of improvement in mental faculties and general sense of well-being. In other countries, the herb has been tested with positive results on proofreaders and radio telegraph workers. James Duke, a botanist retired from the U.S. Department of Agriculture, has stated, however, "I've grown it, and I've written about it, and I went through all of the English versions of Chinese, Japanese, and Korean literature about it. But I remain above all things a skeptic. Ginseng may be good for you, but so are carrots, and they're a whole lot cheaper."

Don't a lot of athletes take ginseng?

Ginseng has been proposed as a performance booster for athletes, and many athletes have tried it. There is anecdotal evidence of its effectiveness. However, when Wayne State University exercise physiologist H.J. Engels, Ph.D., tested ginseng on a group of female athletes, the results were discouraging. For 8 weeks, each athlete took a placebo or 200 mg. of ginseng extract every day.

At the end of that time, each athlete pedaled to exhaustion on a stationary bike and was monitored for performance factors during and immediately after exercise. There was no increase in performance and no reduction in recovery time. Then Engles duplicated the study, this time testing for mood benefit and positive effect on "perceived exertion." Again the result was negative. The subjects did not report feeling better or having any sense that the pedaling was easier.

However, proponents of ginseng say that a minimum daily dosage is 500 mg. They would doubtless believe that the athletes in this study were not given enough ginseng to do them any good.

Would attitudes toward ginseng change if there were a positive study in, for example, the JAMA?

Look what happened to ginkgo. Certainly American physicians and scientist would take ginseng somewhat more seriously if it were the subject of a similarly scientific American study. However, one of the notable differences between ginkgo and ginseng is that the former has *specific* medicinal properties that we are now exploring the significance of. We *know* that ginkgo is an antioxidant and an anti-inflammatory and that it improves blood circulation. The claims for ginseng are usually considerably more general and often spoken of in terms that are unfamiliar to Western science, such as *yin* and *yang*. For better or worse, few allopathic physicians—those involved in traditional Western medicine—are going to prescribe a substance to increase your yin. More recently, some U.S. studies are being done that may change this situation.

Is ginseng safe to experiment with?

It's almost as safe as ginkgo. Indeed, the botanist we mentioned before, James Duke, says it's safer than coffee, although he believes pregnant women and people with high blood pressure should not take it. Other authorities also affirm that ginseng is a fundamentally safe substance.

What is Indian ginseng? Is it another form of the same herb?

No, "Indian ginseng" is actually an herb called ashwagandha, which is the root of the shrub *Withania somnifera*. Its only relation to ginseng is that it has similar properties. Like ginseng, it is an adaptogen and is used to promote calm and balance in the mind and body. Its proponents say that it makes them sleep more soundly and that it rejuvenates them. Its impact on memory, if it has one, would be a result of the herb's effect on the central nervous system generally.

How does ashwagandha work?

It contains alkaloids and steroidal lactones, which relax the central nervous system; and it contains a number of important amino acids, including alanine, glycine, proline, tyrosine, and valine. Presumably, these are the sources of its efficacy.

What is the evidence that ashwagandha improves memory?

There is no direct evidence with regard to memory in humans, but scientific testing of the herb has only recently begun. A study in Germany on male rats showed that ashwagandha affects acetylcholine metabolism in the brain. Since this neurotransmitter is involved in memory and is deficient in Alzheimer's patients, the research indicates that ashwagandha may indeed enhance memory.

One fairly important study has been done with regard to aging in general. Researchers in New Delhi conducted a double-blind, randomized study of 101 healthy male adults between the ages of 50 and 59. The study lasted for a year. The men taking ashwagandha appeared to have experienced a slowing of the aging process. They had less gray hair, higher red-blood-cell counts, and lower serum-cholesterol levels. Three-quarters of the men also reported improved sexual performance.

Does ashwagandha have any serious side effects?

In reasonable doses, there don't appear to be any dangers. Large doses, however, could cause gastrointestinal upset and/or irritate the mucous membranes. Ashwagandha may also increase the effects of barbiturates and so should not be taken with any kind of sedative. Pregnant women should consult their doctors before taking the herb.

What form is ashwagandha taken in and what dosage should I take?

It is taken in a number of different forms, including the dried root, a powder, capsules, tablets, and liquid extract. Two to 6 gr. of the powder or its equivalent is considered to be a standard daily dose.

Are there any other herbs used for memory in Indian medicine?

Yes, there is a substance called bacopa monniera, from the Brahmi plant. It is considered by Indian medicine specifically as a cognition and memory enhancer, although it is used for many other purposes as well.

How does bacopa monniera work?

No one knows, exactly. Little research has been done yet on the herb. It is an adaptogen, like ginseng and ashwagandha, but it may also stimulate the production of serotonin. It has been theorized that it helps to regenerate dendrites, which are parts of the neuron involved in communication with other brain cells. If that were true, it would be quite remarkable, as there is very little, if any, regeneration of neurons in the central nervous system. It will take quite a lot of research to persuade scientists that this regeneration is the case.

What is the evidence that bacopa monniera works?

At this point, most of the evidence comes from centuries of use by physicians and their patients in India. However, one laboratory study on rats showed that an extract of bacopa monniera produced a rather extraordinary increase in learning capacity, as evidenced by their ability to navigate a T-maze.

Are there any serious side effects?

Only if you take enough bacopa monniera to choke the proverbial horse. The herb contains alkaloids, chemically similar to those in strychnine, which can be toxic in very large doses. Large, in this case, means pounds of the stuff.

What are the supplements that provide substances our bodies should manufacture for themselves? Why do we need them?

For a variety of reasons, we do not always produce enough of these substances. The supplements provide what we cannot make for ourselves. Several of them are involved in cognition, some specifically in memory.

What are some of these supplements?

They are the alphabet soups of memory enhancers—DHA, ALC, DMAE, DHEA, PS and Coenzyme Q_{10}.

What is DHA?

DHA, or docosahexaenoic acid, is a polyunsaturated omega-3 fatty acid. Your brain, as we'll explain in Chapter 8, needs lots of these for maintenance of brain tissue. DHA, the most abundant fat in the brain and retina, is crucial to brain development in children and cell-membrane repair in adults.

How does DHA affect memory and cognition?

It appears to increase concentration and improve memory and has been used for a number of mental disorders, such as depression, Attention Deficit Hyperactivity Disorder, dyslexia, and Alzheimer's. It seems likely, however, that it is effective only when there is a deficiency in the body's own production of DHA.

Is the body very likely to be deficient in DHA?

Actually, it is. The primary dietary source of DHA, as well as other omega-3 fatty acids, is fatty fish such as salmon or tuna, and you would have to eat it three or four times a week to get enough. There are no really good vegetarian sources.

There's a small amount in seaweed, and flaxseed oil contains a DHA precursor, but vegetarians have a very good chance of being deficient. Most nonvegetarians probably don't eat enough tuna to keep up their supply of DHA either. In the article we mentioned earlier from *Natural Health* magazine, when twelve experts in the field of cognitive health were asked what supplements they took themselves, four reported that they took DHA. (Five took ginkgo, and the three other most popular supplements were coenzyme Q_{20} and vitamins E and C.)

What form does DHA come in, and what dosage should I take?

You can take fish-oil capsules, which contain considerable DHA, or you can take capsules of pure DHA in sunflower oil. Some nutritionists feel that fish-oil capsules are too likely to contain mercury; they recommend the pure DHA, which is extracted from algae. A recommended dosage would be 100 to 200 mg. After checking with their doctors, pregnant and lactating women may want to take 200 mg. Diabetics should also check with their doctors, as there have been warnings in the past about DHA use for people with that condition. There is also the possibility that DHA might interfere with the absorption of vitamin E.

What about the other alphabet supplements? Do they work in the same way?

No. Each one of them is different and fills a different need. ALC, or acetyl L-carnitine, is a natural body chemical that helps transport fats into the mitochondria, which are the cells' energy producers. Its proponents claim that ALC facilitates communication between the right and left hemispheres of the brain, thereby increasing creativity as well as enhancing cognition.

How does ALC work to help memory?

Some researchers believe that it works with the neurotransmitter acetylcholine. So far, there are only European studies, but this research has shown that adults suffering from mild to moderate dementia may be able to improve their cognitive function by taking synthetic ALC. More research is needed.

Are there side effects?

There don't seem to be any serious side effects, but pregnant and lactating women should consult their doctors.

What form does ALC come in and what dosage should I take?

ALC usually comes in tablet form. A recommended dose is 1,000 mg. per day, usually two tablets. ALC is more expensive than most supplements, up to three dollars per day.

Are there any other supplements that affect the production or use of acetylcholine?

Because of its involvement in Alzheimer's disease, acetylcholine has been the subject of a great deal of research. DMAE, or dimethylaminoethanol, is another substance that, when it is produced naturally by the brain, is important to the production of this crucial neurotransmitter. There is not enough research yet here, either. If dietary DMAE works in the same way that the body's own DMAE works, it should enhance memory in anyone who suffers from a deficiency of acetylcholine. That would include Alzheimer's patients, at the very least. However, there is not yet enough research showing that the supplement can be utilized effectively by the brain.

What is PS? I'm starting to hear a lot about it.

PS is short for phosphatidylserine, a substance that occurs naturally in the membranes of nerve cells. It enhances enzymes that help to monitor the production and release of neurotransmitters, such as acetylcholine and dopamine, and also benefits the brain's ability to metabolize glucose. Like DHA, it can also help maintain cell membranes. In his continuing studies into ARCD, Thomas Crook at Stanford and colleagues at Vanderbilt University gathered 149 volunteers, between the age of 50 and 75, whom they believed to have no significant memory loss other than that related to their ages. For 12 weeks, half of these volunteers were given PS and half given a placebo. At the end of that time, Crook reported, "The group given PS, especially those who were most impaired, improved in their ability to learn and recall names, faces, and numbers. The most memory-impaired among them reversed, in 3 months, an estimated 12 years of decline in being able to match a name with a face." There was another, larger study done in Italy. It had equally positive results.

This sounds terrific. Where can I get PS?

You can't, not the kind that was used in these studies anyway. The PS used in this research was made from cows' brains. After the recent outbreaks of "mad cow disease," this was no longer considered a desirable source. So, the PS you'll find now is made from soybeans. Unfortunately, there is no evidence that it will do what the cow-brain PS did. The only study done so far with it was inconclusive. If you decide to take PS, the recommended dosage is 100 to 200 mg. twice daily. Some nutritionists, however, say that your body can produce plenty of its own PS if you eat the right foods.

What foods help you produce PS?

You need the amino acid methionine, which is found in nuts, seeds, corn, rice, and other grains. You also need folic acid, which is found in leafy green vegetables; essential fatty acids, which are found in fish and flaxseed oil; and vitamin B_{12}, which is found in eggs, dairy products, fish, and meat.

What about choline? I know a lot of people who take choline.

Choline is a substance found in a number of different foods, including egg yolks, liver, soybeans, and peanuts. You can also get it by taking lecithin or any of a number of memory supplements, such as Brain Fuel, BrainStorm, and Food for Thought. Although choline really belongs in the chapter on nutrition, we'll deal with it here because it is so often mentioned in the same breath with herbs and other memory enhancers. The reason it is touted as a memory enhancer is that it is an essential part of the neurotransmitter acetylcholine. Also, scientists have discovered that, by lowering the level of choline in the brains of animals and human volunteers, they can produce the symptoms of memory disturbance that are found in older people.

So, by adding choline to the brain, you can reverse those symptoms?

Yes, you probably could. The problem is that taking choline into your system does not mean that it gets to your brain. Bruce Cohen, director of the Brain Imaging Center at McLean Hospital in Belmont, Massachusetts, says, "We've found that, beginning in middle age, people seem to lose their ability to transport choline from the blood into the brain. Maybe by taking enormous amounts it's possible to force choline in, but we didn't see it with even 3 gr. or more." Furthermore, according to neuroscientist Peter Davies, of the Albert Einstein College of Medicine in New York, "There have probably been twenty-five studies of choline and lecithin for the treatment of Alzheimer's, and the sum total is zero." If it won't work on people with clear signs of dementia, it probably won't work for you.

I've heard lecithin can help memory. Does it?

Lecithin contains choline. That is its one claim to memory-enhancing fame.

What about hormonal supplements? Do they work and what are they?

They may work, but we really don't know enough about them. For one thing, we don't know their long-term effects. And they should never be used without the careful supervision of a doctor. If you already have a normal level of hormones, the possibility exists that supplements could be dangerous. The most important hormonal supplements are DHEA, estrogen, and pregnenolone.

What is DHEA?

Sometimes called the mother of hormones, DHEA, or dehydroepiandrosterone, is a metabolic precursor to the production of a number of hormones. It is produced in large amounts by the adrenals and gonads in infancy and during the peak adult years, age 20 to 30. It then declines with age until, by the time you are 70 years old, your circulating DHEA levels are about 20% what they were at your peak. When DHEA declines, so does the formation of estrogen and androgen in peripheral tissues.

Some human studies have shown that using a DHEA supplement can bring the circulating DHEA in your body up. Animal studies have suggested a lot of benefits from raising this level, including weight control and the prevention of a plethora of diseases, ranging from diabetes to cancer and heart disease, not to mention overall slowing of the aging process. However, these are still just animal studies. *There have not been sufficient studies with people to prove any of these benefits.* And there is no *direct* connection between DHEA and memory. It is simply assumed that if your body is behaving as though it were younger, you will be able to remember more. The same rationale applies to estrogen.

Are there any problems with taking DHEA?

There certainly can be. According to researchers from Baylor College of Medicine, recent studies show that daily doses of DHEA, even small ones, decrease levels of HDL cholesterol. That's the good cholesterol. Decreased levels of HDL cholesterol could increase heart-attack risk. DHEA is also contraindicated for people at risk for prostate and breast cancer.

What is pregnenolone?

It is a natural precursor to steroid hormones. In the body, it is converted to DHEA, testosterone, progesterone, and estrogen. In a study done in 1992, it appeared to improve the cognitive abilities of rats. However, no human studies have confirmed this. Again, we do not know what the long-term effects of taking this substance might be, and it should not be taken without the supervision of a doctor.

Are there any quick fixes? Substances that will sharpen my memory and concentration for a short time?

We really hate to say this. Really. If your *only* concern were your mental acuity, you could fall back on the time-honored combination of coffee and cigarettes. Yes, both caffeine and nicotine wake up your brain. Caffeine inhibits one of the brain's calming neurotransmitters, making you, well, not calm. Nicotine mimics some of the effects of acetylcholine. According to Edward Levin, Ph.D., of the Neuro Behavioral Research Laboratory at Duke University Medical Center, "Several studies have shown that nicotine will improve cognitive performance in Alzheimer's disease patients." Levin also says that nicotine has been used effectively in treating adults with Attention Deficit Disorder and that smokers have a lower incidence of Alzheimer's Disease. *However*, the health risks of nicotine are so much greater than its benefits that smoking is probably the worst solution you could possibly find. Seriously, you can do better than this.

What about memory training? Is there any real value in that approach?

Actually, it's one of the most promising. Like the body, the brain responds well to training and exercise. Quite a number of studies have shown that memory training can improve memory performance in older people, to begin with. One article reviewed 31 studies in which 1,539 healthy adults over 60 were taught mnemonic techniques. A meta-analysis revealed that treatment gains were larger than in either placebo or control groups, that score changes were greater when training took place in a group rather than individually, when sessions were relatively short, and *when subjects were younger*. In other words, memory training was good for older people and even better for those who were younger. In two other studies, it was discovered that the positive results of memory training were still apparent 6 months after the training ended and *3½ years* after training ended. All of the training in these studies was for short-term, episodic memory of the sort involved in everyday life.

Is there any way to train long-term, declarative memory, the kind that comes in handy on *Jeopardy* and final exams?

Yes, there is. The training in this case utilizes the mechanism of memory itself. It seems that we do not store bits of memory entirely in isolation from each other. According to Nobel Prize–winning cognitive scientist Dr. Herbert Simon, "A person builds up vast collections of chunks of memory, and the chunks are then associated with one another." Another name sometimes used for these chunks is "memory palace." "They have empty areas in them," says Simon, "little rooms or slots where you can insert new, particular information. You retain and recall new information that's slotted into a well-known context much more rapidly than you might otherwise."

That explains why expert bridge players can tell you at the end of a hand who held each card in the deck and in what order the cards were played. These are not isolated bits of information but parts of a familiar, logical picture. One of the people Simon has been studying is a man who has trained himself to remember strings of digits, in order, after seeing them at the rate of one number every second. The average person would be doing very well to remember 20 digits. This college student of average intelligence, after training, can remember 100 digits. If you really want to be a memory whiz, you could do much worse than memory training. And it has no harmful side effects.

Chapter 8

Smart Drugs

For some people, the natural approach is too slow, too uncertain. Their focus is not repairing damage to the brain and cognition, but taking normal minds as far as they can go. Mentally, they want to run the triathlon and, like fiercely dedicated athletes, they want every advantage the law allows—and some it doesn't.

What is a smart drug?

The term gained currency in 1990 with the publication of a book called *Smart Drugs and Nutrients*, by Ward Dean, M.D., who is a specialist in anti-aging medicine, and John Morgenthaler, who is a writer. The two had scoured medical journals for any research into cognitive enhancers and put together the information they found in a form that suggested a world of possibilities to its 100,000 readers. With the publication of their book, they acquired a dedicated group of followers who were fascinated and inspired by the thought of pushing the intelligence envelope.

121

Smart drugs, or nootropics, are supposed to enhance cognitive function. Most of them were originally developed to treat memory disorders and dementia. Today, in this competitive society, smart drugs have spread to the healthy. There are reports of tremendous results, including increased alertness, energy, short- and long-term memory capacity, concentration levels, and work performance. A small but significant number of people are experimenting with smart drugs in the same ways that the counterculture of the 1960s experimented with "consciousness-expanding" drugs such as LSD. Indeed, the world envisioned by Michael Hutchison and John Morgenthaler (in "Cognition-Enhancement Drugs," *Megabrain Report*) may sound like a "trip."

Picture this: You have a business meeting tomorrow with your Japanese distributor. This meeting requires that you be in top form for some critical negotiations. You have several reports to go over, many facts to memorize, and above all you have to get some rest. Your first step? A trip to the drugstore, of course. A meeting like this is much too important to take on without fine-tuning your biochemistry. You must create the optimal neurochemical conditions for learning and creativity. You ask the druggist, who then points you towards the shelf of cognitive-enhancement compounds. You load up your basket with bottles of piracetam, vasopressin, Hydergine, choline, DMAE, and maybe a little centrophenoxine.

After arriving home, and taking the appropriate doses of each of these, you go into your study to slip on your cranial electric stimulator along with your light and sound device. You know from your experience and that of many pioneers in the consciousness revolution that this particular combination of chemicals and brain machines has a synergistic effect that will create the optimal psychobiological state for the tasks that lie ahead. You can be sure that your Japanese counterparts are engaged in a similar manner.

After an hour in your study you feel very different. You are relaxed, yet alert and creative. Your brainwave activity has altered, and an EEG would show that it has become more regular and has increased in amplitude in certain frequencies, causing you to feel simultaneously profoundly relaxed yet in a state of intense concentration, loose and creative as well as mentally quick and alert.

A brain-mapping device would show that the two hemispheres of your brain were in a state of "superconnection," with an enormous increase in the amount of information flowing between the hemispheres. At the same time, the rate of metabolism and the energy level of your brain cells has sharply increased. You are now in the optimal state to imprint new memories, to plan new and more creative strategies, to visually rehearse every detail of your upcoming meeting . . . .

Where can I get smart drugs?

If this sounds appealing to you, several smart drugs are available to you, although none of them has been approved by the FDA for this purpose. Their availability is the result of two FDA policy changes. In the early 1980s, largely because of the urgency of finding treatments for AIDS, the FDA authorized "off-label prescribing." That is to say, a doctor could prescribe any authorized drug for any therapeutic use, even if it was not the use for which the drug was originally approved. Later in the same decade, again in the interests of making AIDS treatment available, the FDA approved the importation, for personal use, of any drug that was approved in another country. The approval was limited to a 3-month supply. In early 1992, this policy was modified, considerably tightening up the procedure. In the meantime, however, smart drugs had made their mark. Their proponents can be found on the Internet, exchanging tips on how to acquire them. In many large cities there are "smart bars" where brain boosters can obtain cognitive cocktails—mostly prescription drugs that have been obtained from other countries.

What are some of these smart drugs?

Probably the two most popular are piracetam and Hydergine. In trying to find information about them, we kept running into phrases like "it has been proven" and "a wealth of research." But we found it much more difficult to find specific studies and their results. Its proponents insist that piracetam boosts learning and memory in normal subjects, as well as those who have cognitive deficits. Anecdotal reports once more summon up thoughts of the sixties. "Last year a friend took me to hear Sun Ra and his Intergalactic Arkestra as a birthday present. I had just received a bottle of 800 mg. tablets of piracetam. My friend and I each took nine of the tablets [an "attack dose," they call it in the literature] before entering the hall. The music began 30 minutes later. I found myself able to concentrate as never before. I was completely lucid with absolutely no sense of intoxication. For the first time in my life, I could hear each individual horn's timbre [Sun Ra has about 10 horn players, often all playing massed harmonies]. My friend has worked as a professional saxophone player. He, too, reported extraordinary hearing and concentration abilities. My ears felt as though they were being stimulated from all directions at once, but the feeling was entirely pleasant. I was enthralled."

Neuroscientists are more prosaic. "Nootropics," says James McGaugh, director of the Center for the Neurobiology of Learning and Memory at the University of California at Irvine, "that's the perfect name for these. They have no effects."

Again, the truth may fall somewhere between these two extremes. Research into nootropics is currently being done in a number of areas, testing Alzheimer's patients, children with attention deficit disorder, and normal functioning individuals.

What is piracetam?

Piracetam is a drug that was developed to treat learning disorders. It is not approved in the United States. The first findings on the drug were published in 1971 by a Belgian scientist, Corneliu Giurgea, who was optimistic about its possibilities. In 1976, the journal *Psychopharmacology* published a brief paper reporting on a study of 16 healthy students. Apparently, these students showed a marked improvement in verbal learning rates after taking daily doses of piracetam. Since then, little has been reported about the drug. Unless we posit a conspiracy on the part of the editors of all major journals of neuropsychology, it seems reasonable to assume that the drug did not live up to expectations in this area.

However, in January of 1997, an article in *Biochemical Pharmacology* reported that piracetam does increase the fluidity of brain membranes in aged mice, rats, and humans. This may explain why it is effective in the treatment of learning disorders. However, there was no effect on the brains of younger animals. In another study, published in *Seizure*, in December of 1997, researchers reported that piracetam protected rats against induced learning deficits but had no effect on the control group. In other words, this seems to be another drug that is of value to those with cognitive problems but not to those with young, healthy brains.

What is Hydergine?

Approved as a prescription drug in the United States, Hydergine is said to improve blood circulation in the brain. It is a popular brain-booster drug in Europe and is gaining currency among smart-drug advocates in this country. However, according to Vernon Mark, of the Center for Memory Impairment and Neurobehavioral Disorders in Brookline, Massachusetts, "Hydergine has no therapeutic effect on Alzheimer's patients, and it certainly won't help normal people."

What other substances are used by smart-drug advocates?

There are quite a few of them. They include deprenyl, which was developed for Parkinson's disease; vasopressin, which is used to treat diabetics; amino acids such as tryptophan and tyrosine; and most of the substances we treated in the last chapter. While both the drugs and the amino acids can be useful within limits, none of them has been shown to have any significant beneficial effect on cognition in healthy brains.

Isn't there anything more promising in the pharmaceutical pipeline?

Actually, there is. It's a recent arrival on the scene. In 1996, researchers from the University of California at Irvine announced the development of a new drug called ampicine. It is one of a new class

of biochemicals called ampakines, which were in-
vented by UC Irvine neuroscientist Gary Lynch
and his colleagues.

How do ampakines work?

They are said to enhance memory by improving
communication among brain cells. This is a primary focus of much research into enhancing cognition.

What is the evidence that ampakines enhance memory?

Because the drug is so new, there are not a lot of
studies. The ones there are, however, are quite
positive. Three studies have been made on groups
of volunteers in Europe. The measuring instruments for memory were tests that required the
subjects to remember lists of nonsense syllables,
solve mazes, and recall odors and photographs 5
minutes to 24 hours after being exposed to them.
There was improvement in both younger and
older subjects. The older subjects more than dou-
bled their recall. Even the younger subjects had a
20 to 25% improvement. The studies were done
in collaboration with the Karolinska Hospital in
Stockholm and Cortex Pharmaceuticals, which is
licensed by the University of California to produce the drug.

This sounds great! How do I get this ampicine?

Hold on. This research is really preliminary. The total number of people in all three of these studies is 54. They did not take the drug for any extended period of time. We do not yet know if there are long-term side effects. This is not just a new drug. It is a new *kind* of drug. It will be some time before it is available to the public. Even then, it may be available only for those whose memory has been impaired by disease. Donald Price, neurologist at Johns Hopkins University, says, "It is intriguing. It is innovative. It is worth pursuing. But is it a breakthrough? It is too early for me to be enthusiastic."

Do you think smart drugs will catch on among the general population?

We think that most people are about as likely to take smart drugs as they are to take steroids to increase the size of their muscles. At the moment, there is simply nothing that offers the average adult the possibility of a huge increase in cognitive powers. Steven Rose, head of the Brain and Behavior Research Group at the Open University in England, says, "The big question is whether you could come up with a pill that would cause a 70-year-old to have the memory of a 20-year-old. There is no evidence as yet that any of these drugs will enhance memory in the normal functioning brain of a normal adult. The best that a pill like this could do—if you took it in the morning, you might remember what you did with your house keys in the afternoon."

Is there a point to smart drugs that goes beyond "smart bars" and heightened responses at rock concerts?

In one sense, that's an easy question to answer. The research that is producing these drugs is geared toward curing or preventing the most terrible diseases of the human brain. Scientists are working to find ways to protect the mind and body from Parkinson's disease, Huntington's disease, schizophrenia, and clinical depression. They are trying to find a way to repair the damage done by strokes, tumors, and brain injuries. This is enormously exciting and important work. For millions of people, it could make the difference between life as a functioning human being, with the potential for love and happiness, and life as a tortured soul. In that sense, "smart drugs" are among the most important discoveries of modern science.

There is another aspect of the situation that raises more difficult questions, however. If we are going to have the capacity to greatly increase the mental faculties of certain people, society will have to address a number of important moral issues. Those issues, however, are beyond our scope here. Suffice it to say that, where smart drugs are concerned, there are few easy answers.

Chapter 9

General Nutrition and the Brain

We have been talking about ginkgo and memory very specifically, but let's look at both of them in their own contexts. Ginkgo is effective as part of a general program of healthful nutrition. And memory works well when the other cognitive functions are at their peak. We need to put ginkgo and memory into the larger picture of general nutrition and the brain.

Is there really such a thing as "brain food"?

Absolutely. Everything in your body is fueled by what you eat. That means the health and functioning of every cell, every tissue, every muscle are dependent on what you give them to work with. The brain is a very active organ, metabolically speaking, using about 20% of the energy produced by the body as a whole, in spite of its relatively small size. It gets very hungry and it wants a lot of food. It also wants particular kinds of food.

A Big Mac and a shake may be what makes your mouth happy but to your brain they're just so much junk food, so to speak. What you eat makes a difference in the way you think, so if you're serious about enhancing your cognitive abilities, you should be paying attention to your nutrition.

What are these foods the brain needs?

We're actually just beginning to find out. This is a very exciting time in the study of human thought. The first people to undertake this daunting task were the philosophers. There is one branch of philosophy, called epistemology, that is completely dedicated to examining the way human beings think. It has contributed enormously to our knowledge over several millennia, through the close observation and clear insights of thinkers such as Socrates, Kant, and William James. In the late nineteenth century, the psychologists entered the lists. With the work of Freud, Jung, Horney, and others, our understanding of the mind and its processes began to grow. Now, there are the neuroscientists. Exploring the biological basis of thought, they are expanding our knowledge every day. The Society for Neuroscience held its first meeting in 1971, and some 1,500 scientists and scholars attended. In 1990, the annual meeting drew *ten times* as many attendees.

One part of this new investigation is called nutritional neuroscience, and researchers in this field are doing a lot of studies. Many of them, of course, will take years or decades to complete.

However, some very important discoveries are already being made. Fortunately, most of them accord with what we know to be healthful for the rest of the body. That is, the foods you eat for your brain are not going to stop your heart dead in its tracks. However, there are some foods that are *especially* good for the brain and other foods that are generally considered to be good for your body but are a problem for the brain.

Basically, the brain needs foods that provide the materials needed for the processes of cognition, foods that help with the building and maintenance of cell membranes, and foods that provide energy to the brain. In addition, of course, the brain does best when the rest of the body is getting what it needs. It won't help you a great deal to eat "brain food" if you can't sit up at your desk for more than an hour without needing a nap.

What does the brain need for the processes of thinking and memory?

There are a number of nutrients that help the brain to function better, and they work in different ways. Let's look more closely at the processes themselves for a moment. Basically, the brain is a collection of billions of cells, or neurons, that communicate with each other through electrical signals that speed along the axons—long, thin extensions of the brain cells. As these signals go along, they run into synapses, which are extremely tiny spaces separating the neurons; and they have to get across. The substances that help them get across are called neurotransmitters.

When the signal crosses a synapse, the neuron on the other side recreates the message it carries and passes it across the next synapse, as in a relay race. The process is so fast that thousands of synapses are crossed in a second. The result is that you curl your toes or reason from premise A to premise B or pull a weed in your garden.

That's how the process has been described for decades. Now, however, there is an added twist. It seems that the neuroscientists have discovered brain chemicals called neuropeptides that wash over entire systems of neurons. We suspect that there are thousands of these neuropeptides, although far fewer than that have been identified, and we believe that they make possible the subtlest nuances of thought. Nobel Laureate Julius Axelrod, who works with the National Institute of Mental Health, says, "The brain's electrochemical language is as rich and subtle as that of Shakespeare. And we are just beginning to learn our ABCs." Until we learn more about neuropeptides, nutritional neuroscientists are focusing on neurotransmitters, which are manufactured inside the brain using the nutrients supplied in food, especially amino acids.

How many different neurotransmitters are there?

There are about a hundred neurotransmitters that we know of. Six of them are known to be crucial to cognition, and while they work together, their functions are to some extent specialized. As we mentioned before, the crucial neurotransmitter for memory is acetylcholine. Serotonin is involved in sleep regulation and depression reduction. There are also dopamine, epinephrine, and norepinephrine, which form a group called the catecholamines. They control states of arousal and anxiety. The sixth neurotransmitter is adenosine, and it is involved in maintaining calm. Each of these neurotransmitters has at least one precursor chemical. That is to say, the manufacture of each neurotransmitter by the body is dependent on at least one other specific substance. Serotonin is manufactured from the amino acid tryptophan. Dopamine and norepinephrine are made using the amino acid tyrosine. This is something of an oversimplification, of course. While an associate professor at the University of Bridgeport, Connecticut, I taught a very popular course for 5 years on dietary neurotransmitter precursor therapy. So there's much more to it. An entire book could be written on the production and function of neurotransmitters.

We have already talked about choline, which is used by the body to manufacture acetylcholine. As we pointed out, putting more choline into your body does not necessarily mean that you will have, as a result, more acetylcholine. It also does not mean that all the acetylcholine you have will be used. The functioning of chemicals in the body is much more complex than that. What seems to be true, however, is that by providing the body with these precursor chemicals *when there is reason to believe there is a deficiency* we may be able to bring functioning up to normal levels.

When is the body deficient in amino acids or the neurotransmitters they help make?

A deficiency can be caused by a number of different factors. Alzheimer's disease is a good example. For reasons that are not yet clear, people with Alzheimer's have a deficiency of acetylcholine. If we could get choline to the cells where the neurotransmitter is made, the body might very well be able to produce the acetylcholine that's needed. There is considerable controversy about whether that can be accomplished with supplements. Just putting the choline into your stomach does not guarantee that it will make it to your brain. So far, the best that has been shown for choline supplements is that they can reduce fatigue levels during marathons and similar strenuous activities.

What about the other neurotransmitter precursors?

Again, research indicates that precursors, such as tyrosine, are useful in deficiency situations. For example, the U.S. Army has tested tyrosine supplements with soldiers who were exposed to high altitudes and prolonged cold. In this stressful situation, the body quickly depletes its supply of tyrosine and is unable to manufacture enough of the catecholamines—dopamine, epinephrine, and norepinephrine. The resultant symptoms include memory loss, headache, malaise, nausea, and light-headedness. In the studies, all of these symptoms were reduced by tyrosine supplementation.

So, do you recommend that I take tyrosine supplements?

There are two things to consider before making a decision about taking any of the amino acids in supplement form. First, they probably won't do you any good unless you have a deficiency. And second, they compete with each other to get transported from the digestive tract to the blood. That means that if you take one of them in supplement form, it may reduce the absorption of the others. The result can be a deficiency in one of the other amino acids. You could easily make your brain less, not more, efficient.

Then how can I make sure I have enough of all the amino acids?

The best way is by eating protein-rich foods, which are easy to find in animal sources. Vegetarians will have to do some mixing of foods to be sure they get complete proteins. Either way, you get a balanced "dose" of these crucial neurotransmitter precursors. Choline, by the way, is not an amino acid. It therefore doesn't compete with the other precursors. If you take choline supplements—which may or may not help—the worst that can happen to you, probably, is that you could end up smelling like a fish. It's an unlovely side effect of too much choline. However, you can probably get what you need by eating egg yolks, organ meats, or legumes.

What kind of food helps in the building and maintenance of brain cells?

To put it simply, fat. We've heard so much in the nineties about the miraculous effects of a low-fat diet. It is recommended by proponents of heart health, weight loss, and cancer prevention. It is at the top of the highly touted food pyramid, meaning that we should eat less of it than any other food. All of this makes you wonder whether fat is simply a mistake of nature. However, there are some fats that the brain can't work without, just as there are fats that are crucial to the functioning of the heart and every other organ in the human body.

What kind of fat is good for the brain?

Specifically, your brain needs n-3 fatty acids, also called omega-3s. But let's put that in context. Some of the fats that come into your body as food—dietary fats—are broken down into fatty acids. These fatty acids are used to produce a variety of hormones. They are critically involved in metabolism. And they are a component of the outer membranes of cells, including brain cells. Two of the fatty acids are labeled "essential" because the body cannot produce them itself. They must be supplied directly by the foods we eat. These essential fatty acids, or EFAs, are linoleic acid (n-6) and linolenic acid (n-3). The latter is involved in the development of the brain, before birth and in infancy.

N-3 fatty acids are also important throughout life. As you learn and acquire memory, connections are created between nerve cells. These are the dendrites we mentioned before and they are sheathed in membranes that the brain must constantly renew. It seems, from early research, that EFAs in general and n-3s in particular are the brain's favorite building material for this purpose, and most of us don't supply our brains with enough of them. In an excellent article in *Psychology Today*, Randy Blaun points out, "While consuming too much saturated fat and too much fat overall, many North Americans may not be consuming anywhere near enough n-3 fatty acids for optimum brain health." He cites Carol E. Greenwood, Ph.D., associate professor of nutritional sciences at the University of Toronto, who is doing groundbreaking work on the effect of diet on cognition.

How can I get these n-3 fatty acids?

They are readily available in certain oils—canola oil, soybean oil, and walnut oil. They are *not* present in many of the oils recommended for heart health—corn oil, safflower oil, and sunflower oil. These oils, on the other hand do have large amounts of n-6 fatty acids, which are also beneficial to the body. However, they must be balanced with n-3s or they may cause serious damage. Early research implicates n-6 EFAs, which are not so balanced, with inflammation, problems with immune functioning, and possibly cancer. One study Blaun cites took place at Oregon Health Sciences University. William Connor, M.D., and his team of researchers gave infant rhesus monkeys two different diets. One group was fed a diet in which fat was supplied solely in the form of soybean oil. The other received safflower oil. The safflower oil group had impaired visual development and displayed an aimless pacing that suggested a neurological defect. Autopsy showed abnormalities in brain neurons. The soybean oil group, with no deficiency of n-3s, had healthy brains.

What about fish? I've heard that fish is brain food. Is that true?

Yes, it is. One of the richest sources of n-3s is fatty fish, such as salmon, tuna, sardines, and herring. These EFAs even come in the right form. The n-3s found in brain-cell membranes are *long-chain* fatty acids. The n-3s in fish are also long-chain fatty acids. The n-3s in plant food come in medium chains. It has not been conclusively proven that the compatibility in length between the n-3s in neuron membranes and the n-3s in fish oil is significant, but the possibility certainly exists. It couldn't hurt to give the brain *exactly* the kind of building block it's looking for.

Are all other kinds of fat bad for the brain?

Let's get one thing clear. Fat is an essential nutrient. The body needs it for all kinds of processes. There are only two questions that need to be answered. How much fat do we need? What kind of fat do we need? The answer to the first question is, as you might suspect, not as much fat as most of us get. That's why doctors and nutritionists harp on the subject so much. The answer to the second is somewhat more complex. We have known for a long time that the heart does not like high levels of cholesterol, which is caused by a combination of genetic factors and food high in saturated fats. But what about the brain? In shooting for low cholesterol levels, are we helping or hurting our cognitive functioning? For a time, it seemed that the answer might be discouraging.

There was a huge study called the Multiple Risk Factor Intervention Trial, affectionately known in health science circles as MR. FIT. The researchers who ran the study announced, in their findings, that men with low cholesterol levels had an increased risk of suicide, homicide, accidents, and other violent deaths. This was a serious blow to those who had advocated lowering cholesterol levels as a part of a general program for better health, and they did not take it lying down. They countered by pointing out that MR. FIT ignored far too many variables. They also pointed out the long list of neuropsychological disorders that have been shown to be *strongly* related to high levels of triglycerides. These disorders include depression, manic depression, schizoaffective disorder, and high levels of hostility and aggression.

What's the answer, then? Should I eat a low-fat diet for my brain's sake or not?

Our view is that, since diets low in fat seem to be healthful in so many ways, it would take a very impressive body of evidence to justify abandoning them. The MR. FIT study does not qualify. One example of the kind of variable that was not given sufficient weight is alcohol abuse. Extended alcohol abuse often causes an enlargement of the liver and the increased production of enzymes to process the alcohol. At the same time, the liver increases the production of other enzymes that can result in a precipitous decline in cholesterol levels. There is no reason in this case to look for a causal relationship between the low cholesterol and the potential for violence. There is a causal relationship between the alcoholism and both the other variables. In other words, low cholesterol can result from alcohol abuse, and violence can result from alcohol abuse. So there is no reason to believe that the violence resulted from the low cholesterol, in this case. We cannot say with certainty that the low-cholesterol/violence connection could be explained away in every case, but neither can the MR. FIT researchers assert without hope of challenge that it could not.

At least as important as these variables is the fact that the correlation discovered was between negative behavior and *unusually low* cholesterol. Men over the age of 70 who had cholesterol levels of less than 160 had higher rates of depression, violence, suicide, etc., than men with *normal* cholesterol levels. So, if you're shooting for a normal level, you're not putting yourself in danger, no matter what.

But is there any evidence that a low-fat diet is *good* for the brain?

Oh, yes. To take only one example, Greenwood and her fellow researchers tested out the fat/cognition correlation on rats. After 3 months of eating diets ranging in fat content from 40% to 10%, rats were evaluated using memory tests. Rats who were fed the diets highest in fat and highest in saturated fat performed the worst. Those who were fed diets lowest in total fat and saturated fat performed the best. Mechanically, it's easy to explain. A diet high in fat produces a high triglyceride level. A high triglyceride level increases the viscosity of the blood, makes it thicker. That makes it more difficult for the blood to get sufficient oxygen to the brain. If you want blood that gets to the brain more efficiently, you should try to lower your triglyceride level.

Could I counteract the effects of the triglycerides on my blood by taking ginkgo to make the blood thinner and the blood vessels more elastic?

It's an interesting idea, if you are at the same time working to lower your triglycerides. However, as we have emphasized before, the use of ginkgo or any other medicinal substance to take the place of exercise, nutrition, and medical attention is not wise. It's the worst kind of stopgap. And, of course, if you are working with your doctor on your triglyceride problem, you will want to discuss taking ginkgo with him or her.

What about energy? Is any food better than another for supplying my brain with the energy it needs?

Basically, the brain functions on glucose. The hormones the body uses to aid memory, for example, do their job by raising glucose levels. And glucose is what the body makes out of all the sugar and carbohydrates you put into it. Clearly, in addition to protein for amino acids and fat for omega fatty acids, you need carbohydrates for energy. Simple carbohydrates are converted to glucose quickly, providing for immediate energy needs. Complex carbohydrates are converted more slowly, providing a more long-term, even release of energy.

Does that mean I should drink Gatorade before a test?

That's tricky. In a recent study at the University of Virginia, Paul Gold, Ph.D., and his colleagues gave a group of college students a battery of cognitive tests after having them drink glucose-laced lemonade. Their performance on the tests was measurably enhanced, especially with regard to reading retention. This is one of a number of studies suggesting that a glucose supplement can give you a mental boost for a short time. Indeed, a glucose drink designed for just that purpose is currently on the market in England. However, there are problems with this approach. Depending on your physical condition, metabolism, the stress you're under, and a number of other factors, you could achieve the opposite of what you're looking for. High doses of glucose can cause your blood-sugar levels to go up and then down like a roller coaster. The sudden drop in blood sugar could make your mental performance worse, not better. It may be better simply to make sure your body has all the carbohydrates it needs. The brain gets priority on glucose anyway.

Is there anything that will help keep me alert and focused for a short period of time?

You already know at least one anwer to that question. The neurotransmitter adenosine works in your brain to keep you calm, not on the lookout for danger. This is important because your body and your brain need top rest. You can't always be wary, wondering when the next tiger is going to emerge from the bush. However, if you want to increase your alertness, you don't want adenosine working for you. And what is the most familiar adenosine inhibitor? Caffeine. It will take away your sense of calm and safety just like that, making your brain a cognitive Samurai—for awhile anyway.

What about the opposite? Is there a nutritional answer to the problem of anxiety and/or depression?

Again, we need to talk about affecting neurotransmitters. The neurotransmitter serotonin helps you to feel less anxious and unhappy. Its precursor is tryptophan, and for a long time health-food stores have sold tryptophan supplements to help people feel calm. Now it turns out that the real issue is *not* getting more tryptophan into your body, but getting the already existing tryptophan access to the brain. Judith Wurtman, Ph.D., who is a research scientist at the Massachusetts Institute of Technology, contends that the best way to get tryptophan through the blood/brain barrier is to eat carbohydrates.

I thought amino acids like tryptophan were made from protein.

They are. And when you eat protein, all the amino acids start competing to get into the brain. However, when you eat a carbohydrate snack, *without protein*, the hormone insulin pours in to your bloodstream and begins cleaning up. It begins with the carbohydrates and then gets rid of the amino acids that are hanging around from previous meals, all except tryptophan. Insulin leaves tryptophan alone and it can float right into the brain without any competition. In the brain it is converted to serotonin, and bingo! You feel happier, less depressed, and better able to concentrate.

Are there any particular vitamins that help the brain function?

The B vitamins are crucial to the nourishment of the nervous system. Vitamins A, C, and E are important antioxidants. There are also antioxidants in green tea and red wine and a number of other substances, including, of course, ginkgo.

Which of the B vitamins is involved in brain nourishment? And, by the way, why is there *one* vitamin A, *one* vitamin C, and a whole bunch of vitamin Bs?

How long have you been waiting to ask that question? To begin with, a vitamin is one of a group of unrelated organic compounds that are essential for good health but only in minute amounts. They are a diverse group, in terms of chemistry and function in the body. Most of them, like EFAs, cannot be manufactured by your body but must be obtained through food. (The exceptions are folic acid, niacin, and B_{12}, which are synthesized by your body in tiny amounts.)

There are at least 10 B vitamins, but we once thought there was only one. The first step in their discovery occurred about a century ago when a Dutch physician, living in Java, diagnosed beriberi in a flock of chickens and cured it by feeding them rice bran. In humans, the symptoms of beriberi—which is caused by a thiamine (vitamin B_1) deficiency—are poor memory, irritability, and fatigue, among others. As the years passed, other physicians and scientists built our knowledge about thiamine and its cousins, which include B_2 (riboflavin), B_3 (niacin), B_5 (pantothenic acid), B_6 (a group of related compounds that includes pyridoxine, pyridoxal, pyridoxamine), B_{12} (cyanocobalamin), folic acid, and biotin. Some of the B vitamins were originally labeled with numbers in order of discovery, but we now tend to refer to most of them by their chemical names. Inositol and choline are sometimes included among the B vitamins, but it's not entirely clear that they're true vitamins.

We continue to group these vitamins for a number of reasons. They are found in similar foods and sometimes act together, for one thing. They are so closely related that most nutritionists warn against taking supplements of individual B vitamins, fearing that this may create deficiencies of the others.

What role does the extended family of B vitamins play in the brain?

For one thing, they are involved, along with amino acids, in the manufacture of neurotransmitters. Pyridoxal phosphate, a B_6 nuclear family member, is crucial to the synthesis of the neurotransmitters serotonin and dopamine. Without sufficient thiamine, the neurotransmitters glutamate and aspartate fall into a decline. We've already talked about choline, which is needed for acetylcholine.

What happens if you don't get enough B vitamins?

The list of conditions begins with the classic vitamin-B deficiency illnesses, beriberi and pellagra. Both of these conditions, in addition to physical symptoms, cause neuropsychological problems. They are more common among alcoholics than among the general population in the United States but they can occur in anyone with a nutritionally deficient diet, including those who live in poverty and those who severely limit their caloric intake. Both can also lead to much more serious conditions.

Other neuropsychological illnesses are now being investigated to determine whether the B vitamins are implicated. Niacin, folate, and B_6, for example, are being used in the treatment of schizophrenia. Hyperactive children have been given B_6 to raise their serotonin levels. Physicians have also used B_6 to aid in the treatment of autism, depression (caused by hormonal variations in women), and a rare form of epilepsy.

What if you don't have any of these serious illnesses? Can B vitamins enhance the performance of the brain in the rest of us?

A lot of research is being done to answer that question. We no longer believe that a vitamin deficiency must reveal itself in obvious symptoms or blood tests in order to affect physical and mental health. So far, we have discovered that even slightly lowered levels of niacin may result in depression, a feeling of apprehension, and unusual irritability. A similarly slight deficiency of thiamin can cause a significant feeling of lassitude. And deficiencies of vitamin B_{12}, vitamin B_6, and folate may be involved in the mental deterioration that is usually attributed to aging.

Do you recommend supplements of B vitamins for brain health?

Supplements are one route, and they are the right decision for a great many people, especially those who may be at "high risk" for vitamin B deficiency. The following are among the factors that would lead to such a risk:

- Intestinal damage
- Low stomach acid
- Iron deficiency
- Certain drugs, including cholestyramine, cimetidine, sulfasalazine, phenytoin, nitrous oxide, isoniazid, hydralazine, tolazamide, tetracycline, birth control pills
- Sodium bicarbonate
- Alcohol
- Smoking.

These factors also demand a higher level of B vitamins:

- Stress
- Pollution
- Dieting
- Pregnancy and lactation
- Continued, high doses of vitamin C.

Is it possible for a normally healthy person to get the needed B vitamins through diet?

For people who are making a commitment to truly healthful eating, the complex of B vitamins is available in food. However, there are some guidelines to follow if you're trying to get full nutritional value out of the foods you eat.

- Eat lots of fresh, raw whole foods.

- Eat whole grains, dark-green leafy vegetables, and dried beans.
- Get the freshest foods by choosing what is in season and, if possible, grown in your area.
- Add brewer's yeast or wheat germ to breads, breakfast cereals, and/or salads.

What's the bottom line, then, for keeping your brain healthy?

It's probably this. The healthier you are generally, the better your brain will work. Here are our "rules" for good brain health:

1. Get a balanced diet that provides a reasonable amount of carbohydrates, protein, and fat with a lot more fruits, vegetables, and fish than you're probably used to eating.
2. Sleep more than you think you have time for.
3. Increase your activity level in a way that makes sense in your life.
4. Drink a little coffee when you want to wake up your brain. Eat a little sugar when you want to give it some extra energy.
5. Give yourself an extra dose of antioxidant protection in the form of ginkgo, green tea, and/or vitamin E supplements.

Chapter 10

Choosing a
Ginkgo Product

One of the frustrations of dealing with herbal medicines lies in the number of options and the lack of standardization. If you go into the average drugstore to buy ginkgo, you will be confronted by a shelf lined with bottles bearing different brand names, dosages, and, of course, prices. There are, however, some fairly simple things to keep in mind when choosing a ginkgo product for yourself, ranging from the form of the herb to its cost per day.

What should I look for when I'm choosing a ginkgo product?

First, the label should contain the words "standardized extract," or "contains 24% ginkgoflavoglycosides and 6% terpene lactones." This is the extract that was developed in Europe and has been used for virtually all of the important research done on the herb. Ginkgo that does not bear these words on the label may or may not be as strong as the standardized extract. You have no way of telling. And you have no way of determining your dosage.

Is one brand better than another?

In their basic ingredient—ginkgo—all standardized extracts should be equal, just as all brands of aspirin are equal, except for additions. Some products are combinations of ginkgo and some additional herb, vitamin, or other substance. If the other substance is one that you feel you will also benefit by, you may want to choose one of these products.

How much should I pay?

For the plain, standardized extract the rule of thumb has been about a dollar for a day's dose. That is still the case for many brands, especially the more familiar one. However, we found that prices have gone down since the herb became so popular, and that they vary widely. See the table opposite for some of the prices we found in June of 1998.

What about "designer" supplements that contain ginkgo and claim to have all kinds of other things that are good for your brain?

Just one question. Do they have enough of any *one* thing to do you any good? Let's take the example of a popular supplement which says it is "taken for

Brand	Dose per Unit	Units per Bottle	Price per Bottle	Daily Dose Price
Ginkgoba	40 mg.	36	$13.99	$1.17
	40 mg.	72	19.99	.83
Reach4Life	60 mg	60	21.95	.73
Ginkgolidin	40 mg.	100	22.95	.69
Whole Health	60 mg.	60	12.95	.43
Sundown	40 mg.	60	8.50	.42
PrimeEDGE	60 mg.	120	19.98	.33
Qlife	60 mg.	60	9.50	.31
Walgreen's	60 mg.	100	14.99	.30

Ingredient	"Therapeutic" Dose	Amount in 4 Tablets	Amount in 1 Multivitamin
Ginkgo	120 to 240 mg.	20 mg.	—
Ginseng	500 to 1,500 mg.	225 mg.	—
DMAE	500 mg.	160 mg.	—
Vitamin C	500 to 1,500 mg.	150 mg.	120 mg.
Calcium	500 to 1,500 mg.	60 mg.	165 mg.
Magnesium	200 to 300 mg.	120 mg.	100 mg.
Zinc	15 to 30 mg.	10 mg.	15 mg.
Folic acid	1,000 to 5,000 mcg.	400 mcg.	400 mcg.

stress reduction and improved brain function."
The root "neuro" appears in its name, and its
manufacturers claim that "there is not a better or
more complete nutritional formula for the brain
available either by prescription or over the
counter. . . ." What does this product contain?
Why, ginkgo, an assortment of B vitamins, vitamin C, DMAE, L-Tyrosine, Choline, Inositol,
and Siberian ginseng, just to name a few ingredients. What a powerhouse! But how much of each
of these miracle workers does the supplement actually contain? The table above looks at a selec-
tion of the ingredients in the supplement. It com-
pares the paltry amount of each ingredient that is
provided by the recommended dosage—which is

four tablets per day—with the amount that is suggested by the nutritionists and health professionals who advocate using these substances. The table also gives the amount of each ingredient that is found in a multivitamin that we chose at random from the shelves of a drugstore.

Neither the ginkgo nor any of the other herbals is identified as the standardized extract, *making the amount indicated in the product meaningless*. For many of the other ingredients, especially the vitamins, the dosages are not unreasonable, but the tablets contain considerably *fewer* vitamins and minerals than the average multivitamin. They contain *no* vitamin E and *no* vitamin A, both of which are crucial antioxidants and included in almost all multivitamins. In addition, the supplement costs $14.95 for a bottle of 60 tablets. That's a 15-day supply. In other words, you pay a dollar a day for an ineffectual sprinkling of herbal extracts added to fewer vitamins and minerals than you could get with a multivitamin. And you have to swallow four tablets a day. Not a great deal.

Another designer herbal containing ginkgo offers a list of ingredients a mile long, including DMAE, ALC, and Coenzyme Q_{10}, all of which are mentioned frequently in the literature on cognition enhancement (see Chapter 7). But a quick check of the dosages usually recommended for these ingredients and a comparison with the amount in this particular supplement shows that most of the amounts are downright laughable. ALC, for example, is usually taken in 500 mg. doses. The amount in this supplement is 50 mg. Choline dosages are one *gram* and up, while this supplement offers 35 *mg.* The most spectacular difference between usual dosage and amount included is probably that of L-Glutamine, which is usually taken in doses of 2 to 20 gr. and is here offered in the amount of 75 mg. Even ginkgo, which is presented as the primary ingredient, is present in a 50 mg. dosage. Not bad, you might say. You only have to take two capsules to get almost a daily dosage. The thing is, this supplement costs $30.95 for 30 capsules. If you have to take two a day, your cost is more than two *dollars* a day.

A similar product contains ginkgo, PS, DMAE, and ashwagandha. Again, it sounds like an interesting combination. If, after reading about each of these supplements in Chapter 7, you think you want to try them, you might find this product on the Internet and decide to try it. But look carefully at the list of ingredients and the amounts. The suggested two capsules per day contain, together, only 40 mg. of ginkgo, which is one-third of the dosage usually recommended. The other ingredients? The research studies done on PS usually used a dosage of 300 mg. Two capsules of this product contain 100 mg. Smart-drug advocates suggest 500 to 1,000 mg. of DMAE. Two capsules contain 112 mg. What do you pay? $1.31 for a daily dose. Once again, you're not getting enough of any of the ingredients, and the price is too high.

Are all these multiple-ingredient supplements a poor buy?

It really depends on what you want. If, after

looking at the information available, you decide
that you want to take both ginkgo and ginseng,
for example, there are supplements that contain
both. They are seldom cheaper than taking the
two separately, so their main advantage is that
you have to swallow only one tablet or capsule.
Still, for some people that is an important advantage. We also found a ginkgo tablet, within the
acceptable price range, that contained, as a kind
of bonus, quite respectable amounts of cho-
line, vitamin B_{12}, folic acid, and lecithin, as well as
two amino acids. This is rather a scattershot approach to supplement taking, but not actually a
rip-off.

Shouldn't manufacturers be required to meet certain standards when producing herbs and herbal medicines such as these ginkgo products?

That gets into one of the eternal questions of con-
sumerism. Should we trade off some of our
freedom of access to herbs in exchange for more
government protection against worthless products? This question arises, in particular, with regard to a substance such as ginkgo, which is
starting to gain acceptance by the medical community. In Germany, ginkgo is a prescription
drug. Here, for the time being, it is still considered an herb by the FDA.

What's the difference between a drug and an herb?

That is not an easy question. As we mentioned before, a great many drugs are manufactured from plant products. At what point do they become drugs? It's a situation that is reminiscent of the great Ruth Brown's answer to the question "When did rhythm and blues become rock and roll?" She replied, "When white kids started to dance to it." In other words, the music itself didn't change, our perception of it did.

To the FDA, a medicinal drug is one that has undergone a series of tests that proves, to the satisfaction of the FDA, that it is capable of doing what its manufacturers claim it can do. Without those tests, it cannot be marketed. Herbs do not have to pass those tests. On the other hand, they cannot make claims for the efficacy of their products either.

But herb manufacturers *do* make claims, don't they? Don't their ads tell what their products can do?

Read those ads again. You'll see some interesting wording. "Taken for stress reduction and improved brain function." The manufacturer does not say that the supplement will actually reduce stress and improve brain function, just that it is *taken* for those purposes. Another advertisement says, "Nutritional research indicates a significant relationship between intake of certain nutrients [including herbs, vitamins, minerals, amino acids] and proper functioning of the vascular system improving blood circulation to the brain. [Brand X] supplies these important nutrients . . . ." An ad for DHEA says, "Many books have been written about DHEA. These books contain studies which show that DHEA might be helpful with the following . . . ." Herb dealers can also cite the results of whatever studies have been run and reprint articles written by "experts" about the herbs in question. However, if they want to state definitely that their products are effective in curing this disease or that condition, they have to run the same tests the FDA requires for prescription and over-the-counter drugs.

Isn't there any way to make this process more efficient and beneficial to the consumer?

There are advantages as well as disadvantages in the system. Testing drugs takes a long time and a lot of money. The news is full of stories about drugs which have the potential to save thousands or even millions of lives but which are not available to people who might benefit from them. If herbs were subject to the same regulations as drugs, they too would be out of reach until they had undergone the testing process. So long as a substance is considered an herb, it is available to the general public, and it is up to the general public to make its own decisions. In the next chapter, we'll go into this question in more detail and talk about proposals for changes in this situation. In the meantime, you'll just have to inform yourself and make your own decisions.

But how can I be sure the information I'm getting is accurate?

It's difficult but certainly not impossible. There are a few things you can watch out for when you're reading about any new medical discovery or treatment.

1. *Bias.* Who is writing, speaking, or publishing the information? Two of the doctors who were regularly interviewed and quoted as highly critical of the LeBars study into the efficacy of ginkgo were consultants for pharmaceutical companies. These companies may have a stake in keeping people with Alzheimer's using their drugs, rather than ginkgo; and the doctors may, therefore, have a bias against the herb. Much of the information about herbal medicines on the Internet is presented by companies that sell herbal medicines, and a number of the experts whose articles are cited have ties to these companies. This is not to say that these people will tell lies, but that their bias is something you should know about. Whether consciously or not, purposefully or not, their own interests may influence their judgment.
2. *Terms that are not defined.* If someone claims that a product "enhances memory," ask what kind of memory and what they mean by enhance. If they can't define their terms, don't

believe their claims. In the same vein, if the results of a study are reported without detail, don't accept the conclusions the author draws from it. You should be told how many people were in the study, how long it lasted, what dosages of the tested substance were used, how changes in the subjects' condition or behavior were tested, and so forth. If you're told only, "in one study, 40% of people over age 50 experienced improved memory," you don't know anything.

3. *Oversimplifications and missed steps.* Watch for sentences with "of course," "obviously," and "it just makes sense that." They sometimes signal a place where the author is energetically leaping to a conclusion. The arguments for choline are a good example. Because choline is involved in the body's manufacture of acetylcholine, it's easy to leap to the conclusion that taking choline supplements will increase the amount of acetylcholine in the brain. As we pointed out in a previous chapter, however, this just doesn't seem to be the case. The choline you take in a supplement doesn't get to the brain. So, be suspicious of the "it just makes sense" argument and ask for evidence in the form of research.

If the information you're looking at can pass this three-step test, you can probably rely on it, but be sure you look at more than one source. Often, an overstatement, gross generalization, or misrepresentation will come to light when sources are compared.

One of the best approaches to this question of evaluating information is to find a source or sources that you trust, whether it's a particular writer or a magazine that you think offers a balanced view.

So, what's the bottom line right now in buying a ginkgo product?

Think about what you've read in this book. Think about your own health goals. Read the label.

And what kind of ginkgo product do you recommend?

If you and your doctor decide that you should take ginkgo, we would probably recommend a simple, standardized extract capsule. Adding a multivitamin, if you don't already take them, couldn't hurt.

Chapter 11

The Future

As a medicine, ginkgo is at a crossroad. It could become the next aspirin, sitting in medicine cabinets around the country and recommended by establishment doctors as readily as by naturopaths. Or it could remain in the world of alternative medicine, like ginseng and ginger tea. There are a number of factors that will influence the future of this remarkable herb, including the status of herbal medicine as a whole.

In the past decade, Americans have increasingly turned to alternative medicines for help they had not been able to find in the medical establishment. In a survey done by Harvard University in 1990, one-third of all respondents said that they had used some form of alternative medicine. Other researchers believe that 425 million visits a year are made to alternative practitioners. There are now almost a dozen states in which licensed naturopaths can legally practice medicine as primary-care physicians. In Washington state, insurance companies are required by law to pay for their services. In Seattle, county officials have voted to open the first publicly funded natural-medicine clinic in this country.

The acceptance and use of ginkgo is probably tied closely to the acceptance of alternative medicine. It is unlikely that any organization will finance the FDA testing procedures to have ginkgo approved as a drug, and without that many physicians will be unwilling to take it seriously. Let us take the example of a patient/doctor consultation with a patient who is a woman in her seventies whom we will call Sophie. Sophie has had her mitral valve replaced and makes regular visits to a cardiologist as well as her own physician. The cardiologist, whom we will call Dr. Winters, has prescribed for Sophie a vasodilator and a blood thinner. This is routine for a patient with a mitral-valve replacement. However, the vasodilator makes Sophie nauseated, and so she often stops taking it. Hearing about ginkgo from a friend, Sophie asks Dr. Winters if she could try the herb in place of her vasodilator, or in addition to it, so that she could reduce the dose and perhaps the nausea.

Dr. Winters is an open-minded person and likes to feel that he keeps up with the latest advances in medicine. He has read the JAMA article about ginkgo and Alzheimer's, but he has never heard of ginkgo's other properties. He suggests that Sophie's husband might want to take ginkgo as a part of his recovery from brain surgery, but he tells Sophie to keep taking her vasodilator and try to tough it out through the nausea.

This is not an unusual scenario. For the foreseeable future, people who wish to explore herbal options will continue to educate themselves and to consult those doctors and practitioners who are dedicated to making themselves knowledgeable about these substances.

Appendix A

Alzheimer's Disease Resource List

The following organizations are sources of information and help for Alzheimer's victims and their families. They offer consumer education, research, and support programs and activities. They are also good sources of information for other problems having to do with aging and cognition.

Alzheimer's Association
National Office
919 North Michigan Avenue, Suite 1000
Chicago, IL 60611-1676
(800) 272-3900 or (312) 335-8700
TDD (312) 335-8882
Website: http://www.alz.org
E-mail: info@alz.org

This group has more than 3,000 support groups and 220 chapters in the United States. The website presents a great deal of good information about Alzheimer's.

Geriatric Psychiatry Alliance
1201 Connecticut Avenue, #300
Washington, D.C. 20036
(888) 463-6472

*This organization can help with information and
resources for all psychiatric problems of aging people.*

American Geriatrics Society
770 Lexington Avenue, Suite 300
New York, NY 10021
(212) 308-1414
FAX (212) 832-8646
Website: http://www.americangeriatrics.org
E-mail: info.amfer@americangeriatrics.org

*This society offers a wide variety of services to the
older community, all of which are presented on their
extensive website.*

**Alzheimer's Disease Education
and Referral Center**
8630 Fenton Street, Suite 1125
Silver Spring, MD 20910
(800) 438-4380 or (301) 495-3311
FAX (301) 495-3334
Website: http://www.alzheimers.org/adear
E-mail: ADEAR@Alzheimers.org

*This agency is a service of the National Institute of
Aging, one of the National Institutes of Health. It
compiles, archives, and disseminates information about*

Alzheimer's to patients and their families, health professionals, and the general public.

Appendix B

Physician
Consultation Sheet

I would like to discuss taking ginkgo biloba for the following condition(s):

☐ circulatory problems
☐ headache
☐ vertigo
☐ arteritis
☐ memory problems
☐ tinnitus
☐ diabetic tissue damage
☐ intermittent claudication
☐ asthma
☐ PMS (breast soreness and edema)
☐ SSRI-induced impotence
☐ other (explain below).

_____

_____

_____

_____

I understand that research has shown that ginkgo has the following properties:

- antioxidant
- anti-inflammatory
- aid to blood circulation (vasodilator and PAF antagonist).

I know that research into most uses of ginkgo is still in its early stages, but I also understand that ginkgo has been declared safe by virtually all studies and is classified as "probably safe" by the FDA, unless I have a bleeding disorder or am taking a blood thinner. I understand that caution should be exercised if I have low blood pressure. I also understand that there may be side effects, including mild gastrointestinal upset. I would like to take ginkgo on a trial basis, with these three conditions:

- dosage of 120 mg. per day
- period of 8 weeks
- return visit to evaluate efficacy.

Appendix C

Choosing a Ginkgo Product

Check the label for these points.

One of the following should be indicated:

    ☐ standardized extract
    ☐ EGb 761
    ☐ 24% flavone glycosides and 6%
       terpenoids.

If the ginkgo is combined with another supplement, be certain that there are useful amounts of each.

Use the following formula to compare prices:
Divide single-tablet dosage into 120 to determine how many tablets you will need to take for a 120 mg./day dosage.

Example:
40 mg. tablet into 120 mg. daily dosage = **3**
60 mg. tablet into 120 mg. daily dosage = **2**

Divide that number into the number of tablets in the container to determine how many days the supply will last.
Example:
3 tablets/day into **60** tablets = **20** days
2 tablets/day into **36** tablets = **18** days

Now, divide that number into the price of the product to find how much the product will cost per day.
Example:
20 days into **$8.00** = **40** cents per day
18 days into **$6.00** = **33** cents per day

Appendix D

Memory Tests

Here are some typical memory tests. Average results are listed below each one in terms of age ranges.

1. Read through this list of 15 foods carefully, just once. Try to concentrate on each word on the list. Then take a sheet of paper and write down as many of the items as you can remember.

onions	shrimp	mangoes
plums	tonic water	pasta
eggs	mayonnaise	ham
blackberries	basil	brownies
hazelnuts	zucchini	oatmeal

   The average person 18 to 39 years old can remember ten of the items.

40 to 59	nine items
60 to 69	eight items
70 and over	seven items

2. Look up a phone number you do not know, with area code. Dial it from memory. Then try to re-dial it. How many of the ten digits can you remember?

18 to 39	six digits
40 to 59	five digits
60 to 69	four digits
70 and over	three digits

3. Read this grocery list carefully once through, just as you did the first one. Wait a few minutes and then read it again. Read it a total of five times in half an hour. Then write down as many items as you can re-member.

butter	oranges	milk
avocados	cereal	rice
chicken	gravy	paprika
potatoes	cantaloupe	sugar
strawberries	cake	soup

18 to 39	13 items
40 to 59	12 items
60 to 69	11 items
70 to 85	10 items

4. Have a friend write the last names from the following list on slips of paper. Then you read the names aloud from the list below. For the first stage of the test, have your friend give you the last names, one by one,

in the order they appear below. You try to recall the first name that goes with each one. Then have your friend pick last names at random from her pile of paper slips. You try again to come up with the first names. Repeat this scrambling process three more times. Have your friend keep track of the number of times, out of a total of 30 chances, you are able to match first names with last names.

Stephen Novak	Janet King
George Anderson	Darlene Klein
Maggie Brown	Norma Lincoln

18 to 39	21 correct matches
70 to 85	12 correct matches

(No results were available for middle-age groups in this test.)

Appendix E

Diet Plan for Brain Health

PROTEIN

Effect on the brain: Provides amino acids for the manufacture of neurotransmitters.

Recommendation: 15 to 20% of total calories.

Good sources: Fish, lean meats, eggs, low-fat dairy products, soy-protein foods.

FAT

Effect on the brain: Too much fat and the wrong kind of fat may clog blood vessels and deprive the brain of oxygen. Omega fatty acids, however, are crucial for creation and maintenance of cell membranes.

Recommendation: Under 20% of total calories. About 40% of total intake should be EFAs. Avoid saturated fats.

Good sources: Fatty fish (salmon, sardines, mackerel, tuna), n-3 rich oils (flaxseed, canola, soy, walnut).

CARBOHYDRATES

Effect on the brain: Most available energy for the brain; helps to improve mood and fight depression.

Recommendation: About 65% of total calories.

Good sources: Cereals, grains, vegetables, fruit.

ANTIOXIDANTS

Effect on the brain: Protects from free radicals.

Recommendation: Load up.

Good sources: Ginkgo, brightly colored vegetables and fruit (broccoli, carrots, apricots), V-8 juice, vitamin-E supplements, green tea.

Glossary

ALC (acetyl-L-carnitine). A substance that works with the amino acid L-carnitine to transport fatty acids into the energy-generating area of the cell.

acetylcholine. A neurotransmitter. It is found in reduced levels in the brains of Alzheimer's victims.

adaptogen. A substance that increases the body's resilience and resistance to stress, thereby enabling it to adapt to environmental and other factors.

Age Related Cognitive Disorder (ARCD). Physically caused loss of memory after the age of 40.

Alzheimer's disease. An incurable, degenerative disease of the brain that usually occurs in the later years of life.

amino acids. Protein building blocks, some of which serve as neurotransmitters.

anecdotal evidence. Evidence that is not based on scientifically structured research, but on personal, individual experience.

anticoagulant. Substance which interferes with the aggregation of platelets that causes blood clotting.

antidepressant. A medication prescribed for the treatment of depression.

anti-inflammatory. Drug that reduces inflammation, which is the swelling, heat, and pain that are part of the body's reaction to injury.

antioxidant. Substance that destroys free radicals.

arteritis. Inflammation of an artery.

axon. The part of a neuron involved in the travel of impulses away from the cell body.

beta amyloid. A sticky protein that causes a narrowing of blood vessels in the brain.

bioflavonoid. A chemical substance found in many plants that helps to keep the cell membranes of small blood vessels permeable.

blood-brain barrier. Barrier that is permeable by such substances as glucose and alcohol, but which keeps out large molecules and charged particles.

brain. The part of the central nervous system that is inside the skull. It is the center of consciousness and all voluntary action.

brain stem. The part of the central nervous system that is between the thalamus and the spinal cord.

bulimia. An eating disorder characterized by gorging and vomiting.

cardiovascular. Of or concerning the heart and blood vessels.

central nervous system (CNS). The brain and the spinal cord.

cerebral. Of or concerning the brain.

choline. A substance that is an essential part of the neurotransmitter acetylcholine. It is available in a number of foods, including egg yolks and liver.

cholinesterase enzyme. An enzyme in the brain that breaks down the neurotransmitter acetylcholine to acetate and choline.

cholinesterase inhibitors. A drug that inhibits the action of the cholinesterase enzyme.

cognition. Mental processes such as memory and thought.

computerized tomography (CT). An imaging method that recreates two-dimensional cross sections of parts of the body. X-rays are taken at several angles and fed to a computer, which makes a whole image from the different perspectives; also called CAT scan.

contraindication. Evidence that a substance or treatment could be harmful under specific circumstances.

Creutzfeldt-Jakob disease. An extremely rare disease, caused by a virus, which results in dementia symptoms similar to those of Alzheimer's.

crystallized intelligence. Skills that are learned through education and practice.

DHA (docosahexaenoic acid). A polyunsaturated omega-3 fatty acid that is an essential building block of brain tissue involved in communication between neurons.

DHEA (dehydroepiandrosterone). The body's master hormone, produced by the adrenal cortex and the gonads. It is used by the body in the manufacture of a number of other hormones, most notably testosterone and estrogen.

DMAE (dimethylaminoethanol). A substance that is involved in the production of the neurotransmitter acetylcholine.

declarative memory. "Remembering that"; the memory of facts, names, categories, etc.

degenerative. Describing the condition of worsening.

dementia. Significant loss of intellectual abilities, such as memory capacity, severe enough to interfere with social or occupational functioning.

dendrites. Cellular extensions, generally shorter and thicker than axons and usually regarded as the input side of the cell.

depression. A highly negative emotional state, characterized by despair, passivity, and inability to experience pleasure.

diabetic retinopathy. Degeneration of the retina of the eye that is caused by diabetes.

donepezil (brand-named Aricept). Cholinesterase inhibitor used to treat the symptoms of Alzheimer's disease.

double-blind study. A study in which neither the participants nor the researchers know who is taking the experimental drug and who is taking the placebo. It is organized by a third party.

EEG (electroencephalogram). A recording of electrical signals from the brain. The measurement is made by placing electrodes on the cortex of the brain or on the scalp. The resulting pattern of waves indicates the level of arousal, tumors, tissue damage, and cerebral blood flow.

EGb 761. The extract of ginkgo biloba that is used in most scientific studies of the herb.

EKG (electrocardiogram). Instrument that detects the conduction of electrical activity across the heart. Its major purposes are to detect abnormal rhythms, damage to either heart tissue or conducting fibers, and enlargement of the heart.

enzyme. A substance produced by body cells that acts as a catalyst in a biochemical reaction.

episodic memory. Memory that involves remembering events that have been experienced by the individual.

extract. A substance derived by processing from a natural source such as a plant.

fatty acid. Any one of the many acid chains found in fats and oils; also found as a component of phospholipids in cell membranes.

fluid intelligence. Skills, such as nonverbal reasoning, motor skills, and problem solving, which change and evolve as the individual matures physically.

Food and Drug Administration (FDA). The federal government agency that regulates the manufacture and sale of food and drugs in the United States.

free radical. A molecule that has been deprived of one of its electrons and therefore robs electrons from molecules of healthy cells in the body, causing damage and disease.

GABA (gamma-aminobutyric acid). The major inhibitory neurotransmitter in the central nervous system.

gastrointestinal upset. Disturbance of stomach or intestines.

genetics. The makeup of an organism as determined by inheritance from parents.

geriatric. Of or concerning aging or the aged.

ginkgo biloba. Phylogenetically ancient tree; the substance made from its leaves, seeds, and/or bark.

ginkgo flavonglycosides. Bioflavonoids that are among the active ingredients in ginkgo biloba extract.

ginseng. The common name for the Araliaceae, a family of tropical herbs, shrubs, and trees grown in Asia and North America. The use of its root in medicine goes back at least 2,000 years, to China's Han Dynasty.

glutamate. An amino acid; the major excitatory neurotransmitter in the central nervous system.

glycoside. A compound that contains a carbohydrate molecule (sugar), especially one that is a natural plant product.

gymnosperm. Plant, such as an evergreen tree, which produces a naked seed not enclosed by a fruit, such as the seeds in female pine cones.

hippocampus. An area in the temporal lobe of the brain; the center of declarative memory in the brain.

homeopathic. Of or relating to a system of therapy that was founded in the nineteenth century, and based on the idea that disease can be treated with minute doses of drugs that produce the same symptoms as the disease itself.

Hydergine. A synthetic prescription drug that is sometimes used as a "smart drug."

immune-system deficiency. A lack in that system of the body which fights illness and injury.

intermittent claudication. A circulatory disorder characterized by pain in the legs, brought on by even short periods of walking.

long-term memory. The relatively permanent acquisition of data.

MRI (magnetic resonance imaging). Noninvasive diagnostic test that creates an image of interior anatomy by use of magnetic fields and radio waves.

memory. The brain's record of what has been experienced.

memory enhancer. Any substance or process that increases or restores memory.

metabolic disorder. A problem with certain enzymes or hormones that may affect the speed with which nutrients are processed and the body's energy levels.

mitochondria. The cells' energy producers.

multi-infarct dementia. Dementia brought on by a series of strokes.

naturopathic. A system of therapy using physical forces such as heat, water, light, air, and massage instead of drugs.

neuritic plaques. Patches in the brain that contain a sticky protein called *beta amyloid* and are surrounded by dying neurons.

neurobiologist. One who studies the biology of the nervous system.

neurofibrillary tangles. Tangled nerve-cell fibers in the brain, in the center of which is a protein called *tau*.

neuron. Nerve cell; the main information-carrying element of the nervous system.

neuropeptides. Short sequences of amino acids that function as neurotransmitters.

neuropsychological. Concerning the mental and emotional effects of the organic condition of the brain.

neurotransmitter. Chemical substance released across a synapse, relaying messages between neurons. The neurotransmitter implicated in Alzheimer's disease is acetylcholine.

nootropic drug. A drug that is alleged to increase mental acuity.

omega-3 fatty acids. Fatty acids found in some fish oils; researchers believe they may lower triglyceride levels.

PET (positron-emission tomography). A technique for imaging physiological activity using radioactive substances.

PS (phosphatidylserine). A phospholipid important to the flexibility, or fluidity, of the brain-cell membranes.

Parkinson's disease. A degenerative disorder of the central nervous system, featuring tremor, rigidity, reduced movement, and a tendency to fall. It is marked, in its later stages, by dementia.

peripheral arterial insufficiency. Inability of the arterial blood vessels to deliver adequate blood flow to the extremities.

phospholipid. A triglyceride that has a phosphorous-containing compound bound to it in place of one of the three fatty acids.

phylogenetic. Referring to the evolution of a related group of organisms.

Pick's disease. A rare disorder characterized by literal shrinkage of the brain and causing dementia.

piracetam. A synthetic prescription drug that is sometimes used as a "smart drug."

placebo. A medication that is either completely or largely without physical effect on the variable being studied; used in testing situations to create a control on the results.

platelet. Element of the blood that is involved in clotting.

prefrontal cortex. That part of the brain that controls logic and forethought.

premenstrual syndrome (PMS). A collection of symptoms occurring in conjunction with the menstrual cycle. Its causes are unknown and may be various.

procedural memory. "Remembering how"; memory of a process, usually the result of practice or repetition.

retrieve. Call up from storage, as in memory.

semantic memory. Memory of words that describe things, processes, and events.

sensory register. The instantaneous registering of a sensory stimulation.

serotonin. A neurotransmitter.

short-term memory. Logging of data for a short time.

smart drug. A drug that increases powers of cognition, such as memory and mental alertness.

supplement. A substance that provides, in concentrated form, nutrients essential to the human body.

synapse. A connection between neurons. Most are chemical, involving the diffusion of a chemical messenger (neurotransmitter) from one cell to the other.

synaptogenesis. The creation of synapses that structure the mind.

systemic. Affecting the body generally, as opposed to locally.

tacrine (brand-named Cognex). A cholinesterase inhibitor used to treat the symptoms of Alzheimer's disease.

terpene lactones. Active ingredients of ginkgo biloba.

thrombosis. A condition characterized by the formation of a blood clot within a blood vessel.

tinnitus. Condition with a variety of causes, characterized by ringing, roaring, or rushing sounds in the ears.

tonic. A medication that improves overall stamina and performance.

toxin. Substance that has a poisonous effect.

triglyceride. Fat found in animal tissues (oil in plant tissue).

vascular. Of or concerning the blood vessels.

vertigo. A state of feeling dizzy or off-balance, whirling, or spinning.

virus. A submicroscopic infective agent that can survive only in living cells and that causes many human illnesses.

visual cortex. That part of the outer layer of the main part of the brain that is involved in sight.

Bibliography

Adrian, A. "Gingko Updated," *Nutritional News*. December 1995.

Aesoph, Lauri. "The Facts about Brain-Boosting Nutrients," *HealthWorld Online*, 1998.

Alzheimer's Association, *Web Page*, 1997.

Badash, Michelle. "Alzheimer's Disease." *Health-Gate Wellness Center*. April 28, 1998.

Begley, Sharon. "How to Build a Baby's Brain," *Newsweek*. Spring–Summer, 1997: v. 129.

Bricklin, Mark. "Herbs that Turn Back the Clock," *Prevention*. July 1995.

Brown, Donald. "Ginkgo, A Major Aid to Circulation, Nerves, Powerful Antioxidant," *Health News Naturally*, 1996.

Burton Goldberg Group. *Alternative Medicine: The Definitive Guide*. Fife, Washington: Future Medicine Publishing, Inc.

Bylinsky, Gene and Alicia Hills Moore. "Technology: The Inside Story on the Brain," *Fortune*, December 3, 1990.

Carper, Jean. *Stop Aging Now!* New York: HarperCollins, 1995.

Cowley, Geoffrey and Karen Springen. "Brain Boosters," *Newsweek*. November 3, 1997.

Cracchiolo, Camille. "Gingko Biloba FAQ v.0.1.1," December 1996.

Doner, Kalia and Ralph Schoenstein. "Improve Your Memory," *American Health*, March 1994.

Edwards, Allen Jack. *When Memory Fails: Helping the Alzheimer's and Dementia Patient.* New York: Plenum Press, 1994.

Eicher, Diane. "Gingko Emerges from Shadows," *Denver Post*. November 9, 1997.

"FDA Proposes Safety Measures for Ephedrine Dietary Supplements," MedWatch System Alert. June 2, 1997.

"Federal Food, Drug, and Cosmetic Act," *Title 21-Food and Drugs.*

Fremerman, Sarah. "Clearing the Fog: How to Sharpen Your Mind," *Natural Health*. March–April, 1998.

"Gingko Biloba and Alzheimer's," *USA TODAY*. October 22, 1997.

Gormley, James J. "B Vitamins and Choline Influence Brain Function," *Better Nutrition for Today's Living*. October 1995.

Grider, Katharine and Jill Neimark. "Making Our Minds Last a Lifetime," *Psychology Today*. November–December, 1996.

"Guide to the Smart Nutrients," *Natural Health*. March–April, 1998.

Halpern, Georges. *Gingko: A Practical Guide*. Garden City Park: Avery Publishing Group, 1998.

Hobbs, Christopher. "Gingko: Ancient Medicine, Modern Medicine," *HealthWorld Online*, 1998.

Horvitz, Leslie Alan. "Forgetful Seniors May Thank Smart Drugs for Their Memories," *Insight on the News*. January 20, 1997.

"Hypothesis for Cause of Memory Loss in Alzheimer's Disease Proposed," Public Information Office, National Institute on Aging, May 23, 1994.

Keville, Kathi. "Boost Your Brain Power: Herbs to Improve Your Memory and Mental Acuity," *Vegetarian Times*. March 1996.

Koriat, Asher and Morris Goldsmith. "Memory Metaphors and the Laboratory/Real-life Controversy: Correspondence Versus Storehouse Views of Memory," *BBS*. Cambridge University Press, 1995.

LeBars, Pierre L., Martin M. Katz, Nancy Berman, Turan M. Itil, Alfred M. Freedman, and Alan M. Schatzberg. "A Placebo-controlled, Double-blind, Randomized Trial of an Extract of Gingko Biloba for Dementia," *The Journal of the American Medical Association*. October 22, 1997.

McCann, Brian. "Botanical Could Improve Sex Life of Patients on SSRIs," *Drug Topics*. July 7, 1997.

McCullough, Jillyn. "Increased Interest in Alternative Healing Had Proponents, Critics at Odds," *Gannett News Service*. February 27, 1998.

"More Than a Funny Name: Gingko," *Time*. November 3, 1997.

Murray, Frank. "Learn to Improve Your Health with Amino Acids," *Better Nutrition for Today's Living*. July 1995.

Neimark, Jill. "Opening the Black Box," *Psychology Today*. May–June, 1997.

Netto, Anil Noel. "Health: Regulations Lag Behind Boom in Herbal Remedies," *Inter Press Service English News Wire*. October 3, 1997.

Ochs, Ridgely. "Ginseng: To Take or Not to Take?" *Newsday*. February 17, 1998.

"A Pill That Helps You Think?" *Tufts University Health & Nutrition Letter*. December 1997.

Salaman, Maureen Kennedy. "Mind Your Brain," *Total Health*. June 1996.

Schardt, David and Stephen Schmidt. "Fear of Forgetting," *Nutrition Action Healthletter*. May 1997.

Small, Gary W., Peter V. Rabins, Patricia P. Barry, Neil S. Buckholtz, Steven T. DeKosky, Steven H. Ferris, Sanford T. Finkel, Lisa P.

Gwyther, Zaven S. Khachaturian, Barry D. Lebowitz, Thomas D. McRae, John C. Morris, Francis Oakley, Lon S. Schneider, Joel E. Streim, Trey Sunderland, Linda A. Teri, and Larry E. Tune. "Diagnosis and Treatment of Alzheimer's Disease and Related Disorders: Consensus Statement of the American Association for Geriatric Psychiatry, the Alzheimer's Association, and the American Geriatrics Society," *Journal of the American Medical Society*. October 22, 1997.

Starbuck, Jamison. "Preserve Memory with Gingko," *Better Nutrition*. April 1998.

"Statement by Michael A. Friedman, M.D., Lead Deputy Commissioner, Food and Drug Administration, Department of Health and Human Services, Before the Committee on Government Reform and Oversight, U.S. House of Representatives, April 22, 1998."

Stewart, Walter F., Claudia Kawas, Maria Corrada, and E. Jeffrey Metter. "Risk of Alzheimer's Disease and Duration of Nsaid Use," *Neurology*. March 1997.

Teri, Linda, Susan M. McCurry, and Rebecca G. Logsdon. "Memory, Thinking, and Aging: What We Know about What We Know," *The Western Journal of Medicine*. October 1997.

Tyler, Varro. "Boost Your Brain and Your Libido: Gingko," *Prevention*. June 1998.

Tyler, Varro, Ph.D. *The Honest Herbal: A Sensible Guide to the Use of Herbs and Related Remedies*.

New York: Pharmaceutical Products Press, 1992.

U.S. Food and Drug Administration, Center for Food Safety and Applied Nutrition, *Web Page*. 1998.

"What Are Smart Drugs? A Primer on Smart Drugs," Smartbomb.com, 1997.

Whitehouse, Peter J., Eric Juengst, Maxwell Mehlman, and Thomas H. Murray. "Enhancing Cognition in the Intellectually Intact," *The Hastings Center Report*. May–June, 1997.

Index